Practical
Applied
Roentgenology

Practical
Applied
Roentgenology

Edward L. Maurer, D.C.

Diplomate, American Chiropractic Board of Roentgenology
Fellow, Canadian College of Roentgenologists
Fellow, International College of Chiropractors
Kalamazoo, Michigan

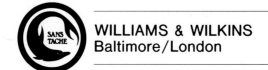

WILLIAMS & WILKINS
Baltimore/London

Made in the United States of America

Library of Congress Cataloging in Publication Data

Maurer, Edward L.
  Practical applied roentgenology.

  Includes bibliographical references and index.
  1. Radiography in chiropractic. I. Title. [DNLM: 1. Radiography. WN 200 M453p]
RZ251.R33M38   1983   616.07′572   82-13566
ISBN 0-683-05650-6

Composed and printed at the
Waverly Press, Inc.
Mt. Royal and Guilford Aves.
Baltimore, MD 21202, U.S.A.

To my family and colleagues without whose urging and support, this work would have never been achieved.

"The important thing is not to stop questioning."

Albert Einstein

Foreword

When one assumes the responsibilities that accompany the practice of any form of the healing arts, he does so with the understanding that he has a moral obligation to both himself and his patients to provide a service that approaches excellence when humanly possible. To become the clinician who can practice his profession in that manner naturally requires diligence not only in the undergraduate days but also in the postgraduate ones.

Educational seminars have been developed by institutions, organizations, and energetic individuals to provide a source of information for the practitioner. Slide-tape and video cassette productions have recently appeared in the attempt to enhance, as a home study course, the learning process. Many methods have been tried to supply the necessary information for the busy doctor, but one explicable fact remains, i.e., that the most frequently used medium of providing informative material is in the form of writings. These sources may take the form of short, concise articles or reports in professional journals or appear as a voluminous text containing the frequently seen material that is of little practical use to anyone other than a researcher.

This is not the case with Dr. Maurer's book. He has accepted his responsibilities as a busy practitioner in the field of chiropractic and as the Radiological Health Consultant to the American Chiropractic Association and performed admirably. In so doing he has recognized the needs within his profession for more clinical textbooks. Fortunately for all of us, Dr. Maurer's awareness triggered his mind to develop this textbook. He had the foresight to compile and produce this manuscript in a manner that would fit into the mainstream of education. His choice of conditions are very typical of the physical ailments suffered by a large portion of the populace frequently seeking the services of the chiropractic physician. The manner of presentation of cases makes for easy reading, and consequently the student and practitioner alike will enjoy assimilating the material. It is done so well that it approaches a subliminal method of learning. The book is not only fun to read but may also serve as a reference text to refresh one's mind about certain radiographic features of clinical findings in many conditions.

Yes, Dr. Maurer is to be commended for his efforts, and it is my good fortune to have known him as a student and now as a good friend and colleague. His never-ending enthusiasm for his profession is envied by all those who know him. I only hope that this text is just the first of many to come.

Thomas M. Goodrich, President
American Chiropractic College of
  Roentgenology

Preface

For many years our colleagues have expressed the desire for a concise, clear text which deals with the everyday problems of clinical chiropractic as it relates to interpretation of roentgen findings. While the practitioner utilizes radiography in his daily practice, he may or may not have retained sufficient knowledge from his training days to identify adequately and quickly a radiological abnormality or to understand its significance.

The axiom "use it or lose it" seems particularly apropos in roentgenology. The student is taught to recognize abnormals and, with the aid of a pattern method of review, to classify the condition into various categories, aimed ultimately at differential diagnosis and identification. Following graduation and with a few years of practice experience, most chiropractors find that they have gotten "rusty" in these determinations. This is due in part to the relative infrequency of presentation of the more morbid conditions, seen for the most part in hospital settings, and also to the extreme concentration with biomechanical variations. This combination eventually leads to a confusion of intellect and diminishes the practitioner's former sharpness to retain, identify, and differentiate.

This text admittedly is not intended as a comprehensive review or a replacement for any one of the numerous, excellent textbooks available. It is written for the non-roentgenologist, for the serious student, and, most especially, for the practicing chiropractor. By design it should serve as an adequate review of common diagnostic problems, demonstrate the ease of recognition and understanding, and, when applicable, provide suggestions for appropriate treatment. I trust it will be used as a ready reference which may prevent a loss of time and be succinct in its presentation.

The cases presented are, with few exceptions, those which have been found in a typical chiropractic facility. They represent cases which might easily enter your office for examination and treatment. I have selected from files accumulated over the past 20+ years a sampling of typical puzzling cases that appear to be of interest to most of the postgraduate students. Each case will be presented with pertinent clinical findings, laboratory findings, if applicable, and the initial radiograph. Specific questions will be directed to the reader which will help to focus thought processes. On the page following the case, the correct diagnosis and other information will help in the understanding and retention of the particular condition. In this manner we hope that an easy, comprehensive, and yet relaxed learning experience can be achieved.

E.L.M.
Kalamazoo, Michigan

Acknowledgments

As in any undertaking, the finished work is in reality the result of the effort and caring of many. I would be remiss if I did not use this opportunity to say thank you.

To my wife, Jean, son, Lance, and daughter, Terry, my apologies for time stolen from you. To my friend, colleague, and mentor, Thomas M. Goodrich, D.C., I can offer only my undying thanks for having taught and helped me along the way. For their cooperation in allowing me the privilege of borrowing from their film collections I wish to thank Drs. A.J. Middleton, V. Muiznieks, A.G. Giambrone, S. Jaeger, E.M. Kenrick, D.A. DeBus, D.D. O'Day, R. Newman, S. Vlasuk, G. Beaumont, M. Gallagher, E.L. Yaple, T. Andrews, and J. Barton.

For their untiring efforts and support in the typing and preparation of the manuscript, special accolades are due my secretaries, Brigita Watson and Mara Skrupskelis.

And my heartfelt thanks to all those who have had the courage to listen and participate in my postgraduate lectures. It has been your comments and interest which have helped guide me in the selection of the material herein. I trust you will find it interesting.

E.L.M.

Contents

Section 4—COMMON ARTHRITIDES

Section 5—BENIGN VARIATIONS

Section 6—MALIGNANT VARIATIONS

Section 1

Fractures

Case 1.1

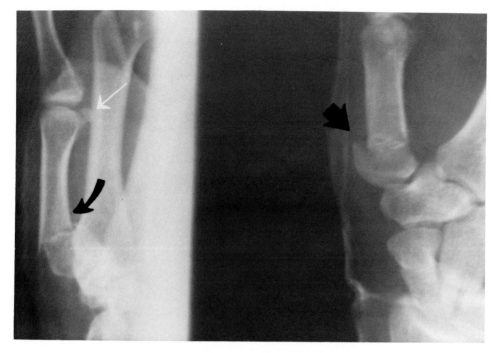

Fig. 1.1.   Daniel S.

This patient fell with great force, landing on his open hand. He experienced immediate pain, with swelling appearing shortly thereafter at the base of the thumb and with accompanying loss of mobility. Is there a dislocation of the carpal-metacarpal articulation? Is this typical of a "barroom" fracture?

This fracture of the *proximal shaft of the first metacarpal* (Fig. 1.1) is *not* accompanied by dislocation of the first carpal-metacarpal articulation. If dislocation had been present in this case, it would have been classified as a Bennett's fracture.

A slight posteromedial displacement (*black arrows*) of the distal fragment is noted, but reasonably good apposition and alignment have been maintained. Note the serrated or saw-toothed margins typical of fresh fracture. The *white arrow* points to a sesamoid or accessory bone of normal size, at its usual location.

This radiograph is not an example of a true Bennett's fracture because of the absence of dislocation of the proximal end of the first metacarpal. It is not a "barroom" fracture, which is more typically found closer to the *distal* end of the metacarpal. In the "barroom" type of metacarpal fracture the traumatic force is against a closed fist, and the second through the fifth metacarpals are more commonly involved (19).

Case 1.2

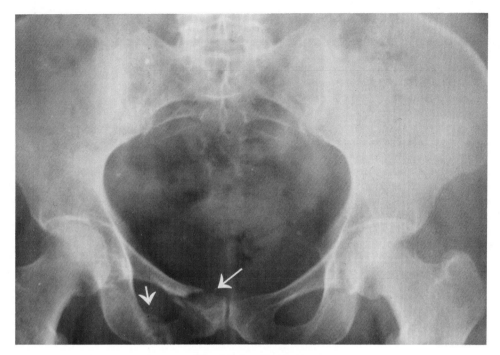

Fig. 1.2A. Carrie V.

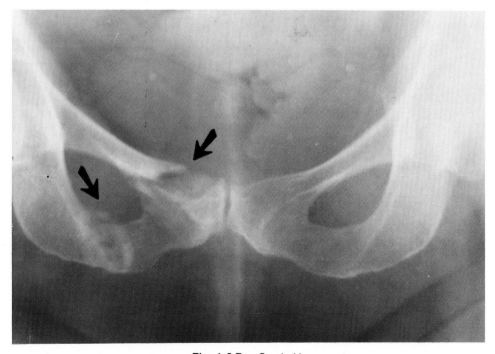

Fig. 1.2B. Carrie V.

After slipping and falling on an icy sidewalk at work, the patient experienced immediate pain in her left lower pelvis and hip. She reported this incident to emergency room personnel immediately following the injury and to two physicians over the next ten days. All reported essentially negative clinical and x-ray findings, and the patient was treated with muscle relaxants for contusions with muscle spasms and allowed to return to work.

Approximately six weeks following the fall, radiographs *A* and *B* of Fig. 1.2 were taken. Rather obvious *fractures of pubic and ischial rami* are apparent on the left. Observe the break in the cortical definition of the pelvic ring and both rami. Close inspection of the site (Fig. 1.2*B*) indicates a good and early callus formation, particularly in the ischium. The size of the fracture clefts and the time lapse since the injury suggest a good cleanup of any debris. Excellent approximation and alignment are noted.

While no dehiscence or gaping of the pubes is noted in this case, great caution must nonetheless be exercised for the possibility of genitourinary injury with or without hematuria, frequently encountered in these types of fractures (19).

Why were these fractures overlooked originally? Some simple fractures take up to 48 hours to be radiographically demonstrated due to the time needed for cleft debridement which will then allow the appearance of the radiolucent fracture line. This case, however, hardly qualifies. All films were later reviewed, and we were surprised to find that in all three instances, only the left hip had been examined! Positioning and collimation had excluded any indication of the real problem. The moral of this story—listen, really listen, to where the patient tells you it hurts.

Case 1.3

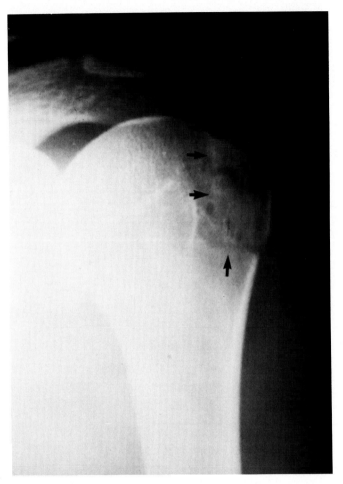

Fig. 1.3A. Tim C.

The patient complained of pain and difficulty in elevating the left shoulder, following an auto accident. Would you expect any difficulty in healing or any residual deformity?

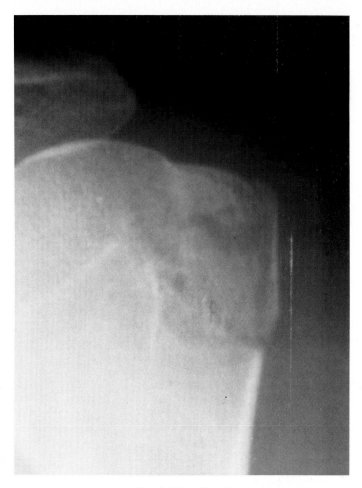

Fig. 1.3B. Tim C.

As in all fractures, interruption of architectural integrity and loss of cortical definition are important radiographic findings. The degree of apposition and alignment of the fracture fragment(s) with the host bone will determine the degree and deformity after healing.

In this case, healing was uncomplicated, with no significant deformity. Treatment was aimed primarily at immobilization to maintain good apposition.

The *arrows* shown on the radiograph (Fig. 1.3A) outline the fracture line which closely follows the medial margin of the *greater tubercle*. Due to muscular attachments on the greater tubercle, this rather clean fracture would suggest a possible avulsion etiology.

Case 1.4

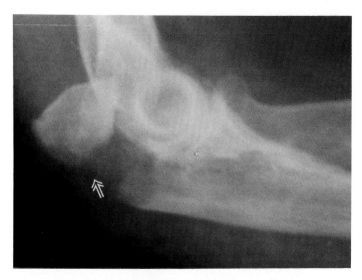

Fig. 1.4A. Neida G.

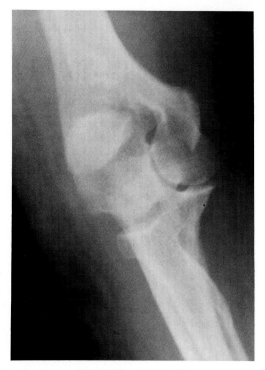

Fig. 1.4B. Neida G.

This 68-year-old woman fell on a cement sidewalk, injuring her right elbow. Being a bit stubborn, she refused to have anyone look at it until nearly two weeks later. The clinical presentation was of moderate swelling over the posterior surface of the right olecranon, point tenderness and inability to adequately flex and extend the elbow. Fig 1.4A demonstrates *posterior-superior displacement of the olecranon process*, now a free fracture fragment.

Because of the effect on function to the triceps brachii, the ulnar collateral and posterior ligaments which attach to this process, this type of fracture should be surgically pinned as soon as possible. In this case, due to the reticence of the patient and the fact that she was left-handed, all suggestions of surgery were refused. Limitation of functionability of the elbow and forearm was a permanent result, albeit adequate for her age and activity.

Case 1.5

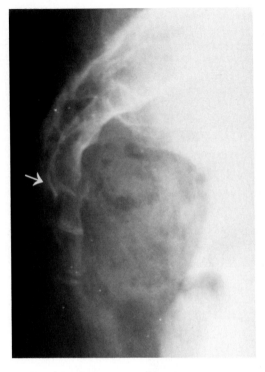

Fig. 1.5. Harriet Z.

This 51-year-old woman slipped on the ice, falling on her buttock. Immediate pain was noted as being low—towards the tail-bone—with an odd rectal sensation. A severe headache with transient nausea occurred shortly after the fall but dissipated spontaneously in a few hours.

The routine AP pelvis film was negative for fracture. The lateral projection (Fig. 1.5) adequately reveals a *transverse fracture* line with slight anterior displacement of the *distal sacrum*.

As this film was taken within six hours of the fall, the thin semicircular markings at both anterior and posterior margins of the fracture line represent either fracture debris or bony margins seen en face. It cannot as yet be callus formation due to the time factor.

The odd rectal sensation was probably due to the force of the concussion with resultant soft-tissue insult. No rectal bleeding was found. Headache and nausea is not uncommon in posttraumatic concussion of the central nervous system due to shock, in this case of the sacral and pudendal plexus as well as the filum terminale.

The normal sacral contour will frequently disallow for good visualization of fracture on the AP view. It is necessary for the beam of the x-ray to enter through the fracture line, thus calling for tube angulation. In some instances it is sufficient to take a PA sacral film to take advantage of the resultant magnification. When viewing the sacrum or coccyx on any film, it is necessary to be certain that no break in contour or continuity is present. Careful review is a must.

Case 1.6

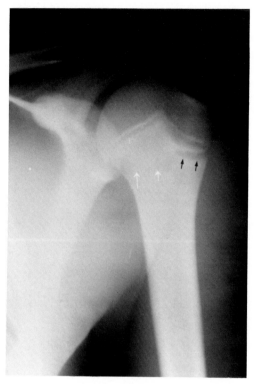

Fig. 1.6. Timmy K.

Tim is almost 12 years old. Two days ago he was "gang blocked" while playing football. Someone's helmet rammed his shoulder in the pile up. Ever since, his shoulder has been painful, even though he is still able to perform full range of motion. Moderate soft-tissue swelling is present, and there is only suggested discoloration.

When rest and hot packs did not relieve the pain, Tim's mother brought him in for examination.

We are anxious to know your answers to the following questions after you review this film: Is the humeral epiphysis intact, is it fractured, is this a complicated lesion, will healing be delayed or result in deformity?

Remember that the typical epiphyseal plate is rarely multileveled. Typically it is irregular in appearance. With injury, it can be separated or fractured, a condition referred to as epiphysiolysis (19). When this happens, variations of the growth plate are encountered which may result in deformity or alteration of the modeling process. A sometimes nasty problem indeed!

In Tim's case, a *simple fracture* cleft is seen (*black arrows*) which closely follows the epiphyseal plate line but which does not interrupt the epiphysis. With careful examination (*white arrows*) it can be detected that a hairline continuation of the fracture line extends nearly to the opposite cortex. There is no significant displacement or loss of continuity or apposition, and the capital epiphysis has not "slipped." This case healed spontaneously, without complication or deformity, with simple immobilization. No sequelae developed.

Case 1.7

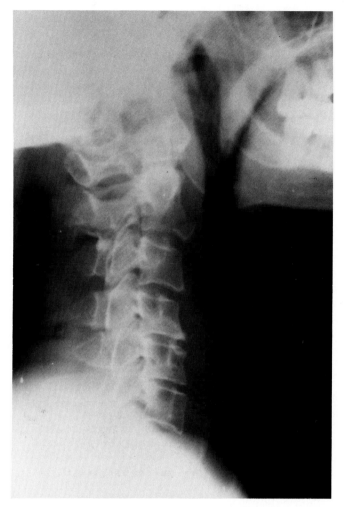

Fig. 1.7A. Nathan K.

This 43-year-old man was having a marvelous time at a friend's birthday party. Having loosed his otherwise timid personality with the help of several martinis, he decided it was a good time for a dip in the pool. Unfortunately he chose to dive in the shallow end!

He was seen at the emergency room where a moderate concussion was diagnosed, and treatment for superficial lacerations, abrasions and contusions was given. He was admitted overnight for observation. Skull x-rays were negative.

Two days after discharge his head was feeling better, but his neck was extremely stiff and painful in motion. Your examination, although somewhat limited due to paraspinal muscle splinting, was essentially unremarkable. Knowing the history, you elected to repeat the radiographs of his neck, including range of motion studies. You see both the acute lesion as well as preexisting alterations. What is your diagnosis(s), and how should you approach treatment for the acute lesion?

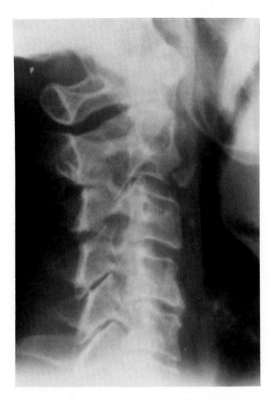

Fig. 1.7*B.* Nathan K.

Antalgic rigidity or flattening of the cervical lordosis due to pain is noted in the neutral view. Moderate discal thinning is noted from C4 through C6 with early discogenic spondylosis. Hypomobility and fixation are noted from C4 to C6 but are undoubtedly due to these preexisting alterations. The amount of osteophytic spur intrusion into the intervertebral foramina at C4–C5 and C5–C6 has produced some foraminal encroachment, but neurovascular entrapment is problematical.

The acute problem is of course an *avulsion or chip fracture* from the anterior portion of the inferior body of C2. Slight anterior and inferior displacement is seen of the fracture fragment, but it appears well anchored within the anterior ligamentous structures. Further excursion is doubtful. There is minimal widening of the retropharyngeal soft-tissue interspace between the anterior margin of C2 and the posterior wall of the air-filled pharynx. This finding(s) suggests the presence of a soft-tissue hematoma.

Treatment is purely symptomatic in that no surgical intervention is required and no conservative approach will significantly improve the apposition and alignment of the fragment with the host bone. Utilization of a cervical collar provides comfort, as does use of various modalities to enhance soft-tissue healing. Manipulation at this time is contraindicated, as this fracture involves the ligamentous attachments of both the anterior longitudinal ligament as well as the anulus fibrosus and has broken through the inferior body plate margin. In time, the development of spondylosis at this level would not be an uncommon sequela. When this is coupled with the preexisting spondylosis at C4–C6, the patient will present with a very unstable neck in years to come, with additional disturbance of cervical rhythm.

Case 1.8

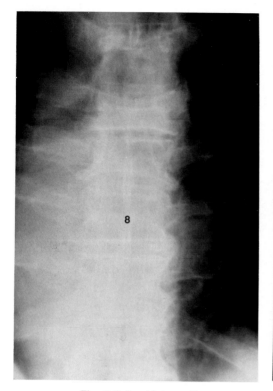

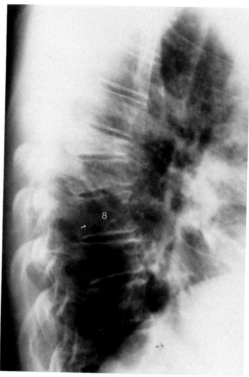

Fig. 1.8 A.   Malcom T.   **Fig. 1.8 B.**   Malcom T.

This 56-year-old Caucasian man reported to the clinic complaining of chronic, recurrent ache of his midthoracic spine. His history included a fall from a scaffold some years ago, for which he had not sought any treatment. His pain at the time had "laid him up for two to three weeks," after which he returned to work as a house painter.

As you review *any* film, you must carefully delineate all margins, inspect the cortices, trabecular patterns, interarticular joint spacing, and all anatomical landmarks. This careful review must be done on *all* structures seen on the film. Opposing views are always taken, as the mini-

mum study, so full evaluation is possible.

In reviewing Malcolm's films, it is obvious that a *compression-type fracture* has occurred at T6 with resultant trapezoidal configuration of the vertebral body from anterior to posterior. Have you noticed also the concave impression of the inferior body plate margin of T7 on the AP view with decrease in the vertebral height? Close inspection of the lateral view of T7 also indicates decrease in vertebral height and a concave impression of its inferior body plate margin near its anterior one third. This indicates prior plate infraction, presumably occurring simultaneously with the injury to T6.

Case 1.9

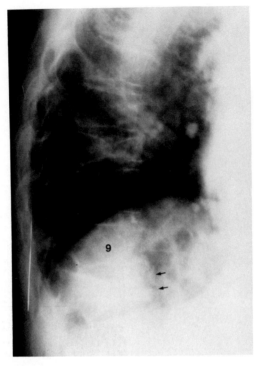

Fig. 1.9. Walter Z.

Ironically, Walter is also a house painter (is it really that hazardous?).

Walter also fell from a ladder, some six or seven weeks ago. His history indicates that over the past 10 to 15 years he had fallen numerous times. (He depended on his chiropractor to keep him on the job!)

By the careful review which was detailed in our last case, you should have picked up the *butterfly appearance* of the T7 vertebral body. This resulted from a *central compression fracture* of the vertebral body with slight forward displacement of its anterior one half. Notice the elongated appearance from anterior to posterior by comparison with those above and below. Careful inspection will identify reactive change at the fracture cleft, presumably an attempt at callus formation and attending debridement of fracture debris. This later finding when coupled with the history is often helpful in determining the vintage of the fracture.

At the *arrows* in Fig. 1.9, note the compression-type fracture with resultant trapezoidal configuration of the T10 vertebral body. This represents an old, healed lesion not related to his most recent fall (trust me!). Have you noticed the rather marked hyperextension of the T10 segment? Notice also the alteration of the T9–T10 and to a lesser extent the T10–T11 intervertebral foramina. Neurovascular entrapment is possible, but altered biomechanical rhythm of the posterior articulating facets is certain.

This film suggests that in time, due to the prior traumatic experience, accelerated discal degeneration will occur between T6 and T7, T7 and T8, T9 and T10 and T10 and T11 (8).

Case 1.10

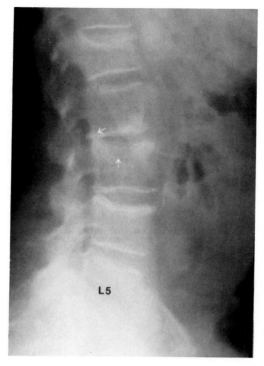

Fig. 1.10. Roger T.

Roger T. has a history of long-standing lumbar discomfort, stiffness on awakening, and inability to sit for prolonged periods of time.

He reports chronic constipation and periodic kidney infection.

Historically, Roger fell 12 feet from a roof some eight years ago. He was hospitalized for two weeks at the time and has suffered periodically since.

He has had noticeably more lumbar pain following a motorcycle hill climb which he participated in a week ago.

With this case you won't have to turn the page to compare conclusions. Roger's history explains a lot.

The body end-plate margins from L1 through L4 present with indentation and concave impression characteristic of *discal impressions(s)*. The L1 segment is trapezoidal with the anterior height of the body less than the posterior height. This, com-
bined with the superior plate impression, is typical of prior compression fracture. The narrowed disc space between L2 and L3, coupled with the *plate infraction (lower arrow)* and the small posterior osteophyte *(upper arrow)*, suggests posttraumatic discogenic spondylosis. Notice the marginal indentation of the anterior-inferior portion of the L2 body as well. This finding is suggestive of a possible "buckle type" fracture which has since healed with resultant deformity.

The neurovascular involvement due to foraminal intrusion by the osteophyte between L2 and L3 is of probable significance in the visceral complaints reported.

Roger's hill climbing had produced an acute myofascial strain which accounted for his acute condition. The overall radiographic impression is one of chronic hypomobility and fixation of the lumbar spine.

Case 1.11

Case 1.12

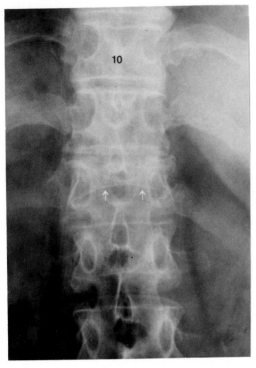

Fig. 1.11   John C.

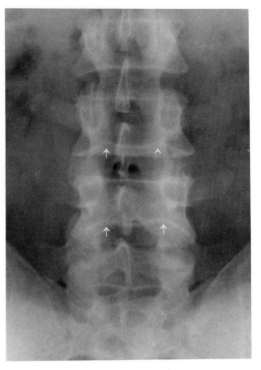

Fig. 1.12   Lloyd B.

CASE 1.11: COMPRESSION FRACTURE

Notice the fine-line curvilinear concavity extending the entire width of the T12 segment. This finding suggests that a trapezoidal vertebral body is to be expected when viewing the lateral film.

Most trapezoidal or wedge-like vertebral deformities follow compression fracture but are also frequently seen following pathological compression, i.e., tubercular spondylitis, infectious spondylitis and eosinophilic granuloma.

CASE 1.12: PLATE INFRACTION

The concavities of the inferior body plate margins (*arrows*) do not involve the entire width of the segment. In this case their location is on either side of the midline at two levels, L3 and L4. When seen, they represent prior compression failure of the vertebral end plates with discal intrusion (26) often predisposing to accelerated discal aging (27).

They are not to be confused with Schmorl's nodes which are usually associated with discal invagination into the thinned portion of the end plate at the remnant notocord site. These are usually located at midline on the AP view but are best demonstrated on the lateral projection.

When interruption of the fine curvilinear margin is noted or if any continuity is lacking, a recent plate infarction is suspect, and laminography may be needed for confirmation. These are not always bilateral.

Case 1.13

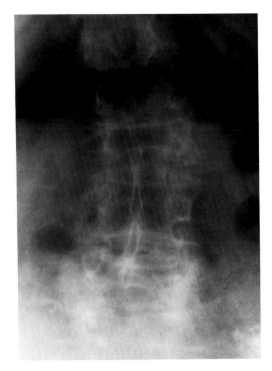

Fig. 1.13 A. Cleo W.

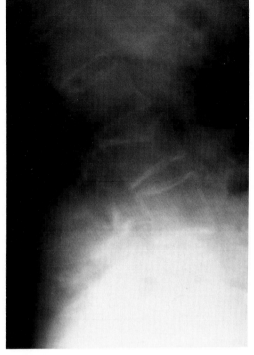

Fig. 1.13 B. Cleo W.

Cleo is an 83-year-old wonder. She is consistently on the go, doing more work in one day than her children do in three. "Sturdy stock" is the commonly used phrase to describe her physical prowess.

Alas, six weeks ago she experienced sharp pain in the lower back while carrying in fire wood. Although the pain was intense for the first two or three days, it has now lessened. A steady, dull ache is reported, as are occasional sharp twinges with certain rotations of the trunk.

Moderate paraspinal muscular splinting is noted with point tenderness located at L2-L3. Radiographs are ordered.

In Fig. 1.13, *A* and *B*, Cleo's lumbar spine can barely be seen. The radiographic detail is lost primarily due to moderately severe *osteoporosis* throughout. Notice the vertebral margin accentuation when compared to the body. This finding is of course not unusual in the geriatric patient.

Moderate wedging is seen on the AP film of L3. The lateral confirms a *compression fracture deformity* of the superior body plate margin of L3, near its centrum. Healing will occur spontaneously over a long period of time, but Cleo's heavy duties have now been restricted. Much relief is afforded during the healing phase with soft-tissue goading and gentle manipulation above and below the lesion.

In the demineralization of osteoporosis the internal integrity and strength of the supportive structure in bone is decreased. Thus its ability to handle stress is diminished. Pathological fracture is common.

Case 1.14

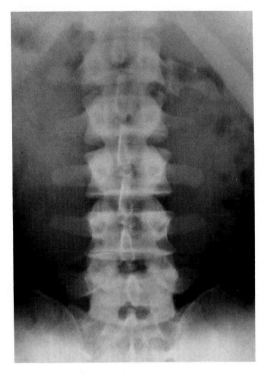

Fig. 1.14A. Juan G.

The question often is asked, "How do you tell the difference between a *persistent apophysis* and a *fracture* of the transverse process?"

Juan was thrown from a snowmobile about ten days ago. After the contusion and swelling lessened, he was still concerned by the nagging pain.

Your attention is immediately drawn to the base of the L1 transverse process on the right (Fig. 1.14A). The fracture cleft is well seen with irregular margination and dense reactive sclerosis. No significant displacement is seen, and healing will progress completely. At the *arrow* is Fig 1.14B can be seen a slight separation of the base of the transverse process on the left. This continues along a line through the entire transverse process. (Its fine-line character was lost by photographic replication.) The distal portion is separated at the base; a persistent apophysis. It is characteristically seen with smooth margins and no reactive sclerosis. Even most ununited fractures retain their marginal irregularity and sclerosis for long periods. The key words are: ragged margins, fracture; smooth margins, persistent apophysis.

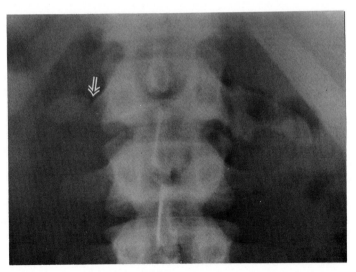

Fig. 1.14B. Juan G.

Section 2

Developmental Variations

Case 2.1

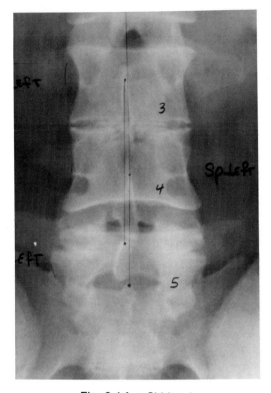

Fig. 2.1A. Shirley J.

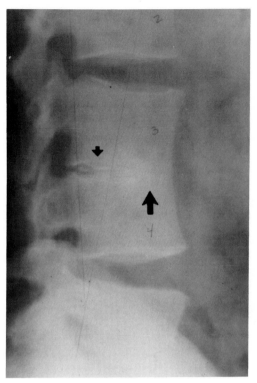

Fig. 2.1B. Shirley J.

Block vertebrae are not uncommon. They are generally found accidentally in pursuit of some other problem. If, on the other hand, they represent ankylosis, the result of some prior infectious process, or surgical arthrodesis, their clinical significance is of utmost importance. Can you tell the difference? In this case would you anticipate neurovascular entrapment?

Case 2.1 demonstrates a *block vertebra* formation between L3 and L4. Note the rudimentary disc space which is present within the posterior one half of the segment (Fig. 2.1B). Calcification can be seen within this intervertebral disc (IVD). The anterior one half of these two segments presents nonsegmentation and therefore has created a solid anomalous segment.

This lack of segmentation or differentiation is typical of most block vertebrae and is the result of aberrant embryological development (23).

You will note patency of the attending intervertebral foramen. This ensures appropriate transmission of the neurovascular structures. Fusion or nonsegmentation of a block vertebra will preclude mobility of the anterior and posterior portions of the motor unit involved. The lack of reactive sclerosis within the involved segments above and below the normal location of the IVD can often help to rule out prior infectious processes. The normal architectural markings of contiguous structures is also an important finding, as is the historical evidence presented clinically.

Case 2.2

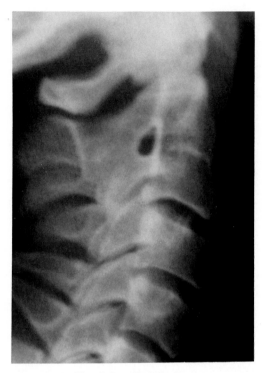

Fig. 2.2. Christie P.

The size and shape of the attending intervertebral foramen (IVF) must be examined. In a true congenital or developmental anomalous block vertebra, the IVF will present as somewhat ovoid in appearance, as seen in Figs. 2.1*B* and 2.2. Following pathological fusion the IVF tends to be shortened in its height with a somewhat "squat" appearance. In the postsurgical case the IVF will appear more rounded or circular in shape.

In Case 2.1 of *block vertebrae*, seen between C2 and C3, the anterior rudimentary disc space and ovoid appearance of the intervertebral foramen is well visualized. Notice also the bony fusion of the zygapophyseal articulation. This nonsegmentation of both the anterior and posterior motor unit is not uncommon in block vertebrae. The remaining cervical segments are anatomically normal.

Case 2.3

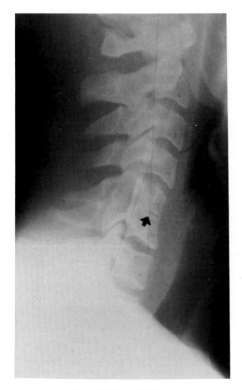

Fig. 2.3A. Shirley J. #2

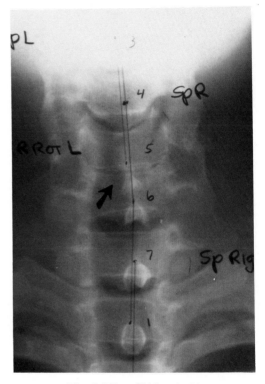

Fig. 2.3B. Shirley J. #2

Case 2.3 is another example of a *block vertebra*. As we mentioned, these are not uncommon. This case is a bit unusual in that the block vertebra of the lumbar spine in Fig. 2.1 and the block vertebra in Fig. 2.3 are both in the same patient!

The findings of rudimentary disc, non-segmentation, and patency of the attending IVF are apparent. Also visible in this case is an extremely narrowed zygapophyseal articulation between C5 and C6, bilaterally.

Often when a block vertebra is seen in the cervical spine, the tendency is to label it as the Klippel-Feil syndrome. This is *incorrect*. The syndrome of Klippel-Feil refers to a combination of block vertebra, cleft vertebra and hemivertebra with associated defects in the neural arches. Clinically the neck appears shortened and wide with a low hairline. Occasionally it is combined with other anomalies as well (23).

Case 2.4

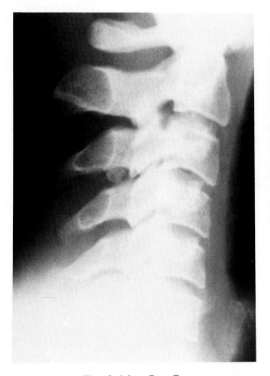

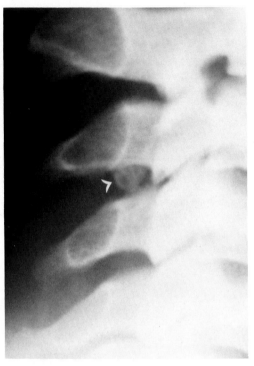

Fig. 2.4A. Don R.

Fig. 2.4B. Don R.

Accessory bones and certain centers of ossification that fail to unite are frequently found in the skeleton. When seen developing within a tendon, they are referred to as sesamoid bones. When representing either unfused growth centers or an accessory bone not normally found in the skeleton, they are termed supernumerary ossicles (23).

Accessory ossicles of the foot, ankle, wrist and hand are most common. A few are frequent in the knee, hip, elbow and shoulder.

They may be mistaken for fracture or pathology if one is not aware of the common site of appearance. In addition, careful examination will indicate smooth margination, intact cortex and, typically, some trabeculation. A fracture fragment will usually present with irregular margination.

In Don's case (Fig. 2.4, *A* and *B*), a well-marginated bony structure is seen between the spinous processes of C3 and C4. It lies anterior of the laminaspinous process junction. Were it to be located at midline, production of vertebral canal stenosis would be expected. The AP radiograph does confirm that it is situated lateral to the spine, within the soft tissues—an incidental finding.

Accessory bones are rarely of clinical importance. This case is included due to its rather unusual location and appearance.

Do not confuse the joint "mouse" which results from pathological fragmentation and/or formation, or a fracture, with the normal accessory or supernumerary ossicle.

Case 2.5

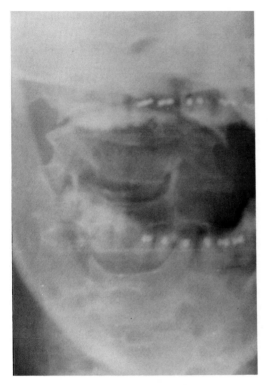

Fig. 2.5A. Nancy D.

Nancy had had headache with some stiffness at the base of the skull for a long time. There had been no significant history of trauma.

More recently the stiffness had become more noticeable, and constant fatigue had been noted in the atlantooccipital region.

Her new job as a receptionist required her to spend a great deal of time on the telephone. She admitted she had a habit of cradling the receiver between the head and shoulder.

Our question to you is threefold. First, can you identify the lesion responsible for her present complaint? Next, is it congenital, traumatic or pathological? Lastly, is manipulation contraindicated?

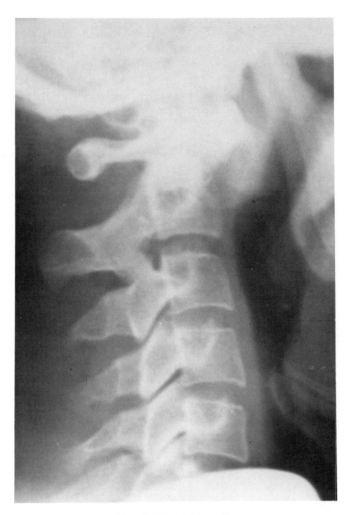

Fig. 2.5B. Nancy D.

The lateral view (Fig. 2.5B) shows definite forward displacement of the head and neck above C2. This is most unusual unless the transverse ligament of C1 has been torn by injury. Nancy had had no such history. The degree of right lateral listhesis of C1 on C2 is dramatic, as seen in Fig. 2.5A. By this time you should have noticed that what you took for the odontoid process on the AP open mouth view has its base well below the superior margin of C2. In reality you have identified a tooth. This patient has a complete *agenesis* or absence *of the odontoid process.*

While this finding is developmental in origin, it nonetheless represents a significant biomechanical variation. The entire atlantooccipital rhythm and stability are totally dependent on ligamentous integrity. While manipulation is not contraindicated, it must be done in a gentle fashion to stay within the limits of the musculoligamentous tolerance. The recent symptoms are related to the positional disrelationship between C1 and C2 and C2 and C3, coupled with postural stress and/or fatigue associated with her new job. A telephone shoulder cradle was suggested.

Case 2.6

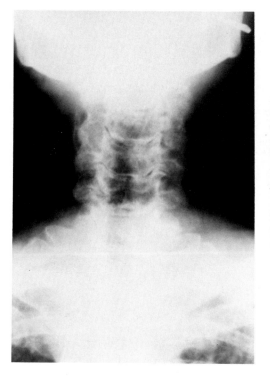

Fig. 2.6A. Ida S.

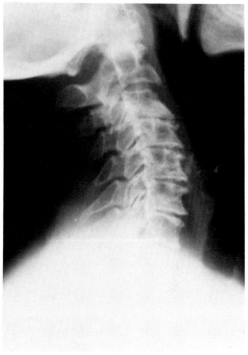

Fig. 2.6B. Ida S.

This 70-year-old woman (Fig. 2.6, A and B) reports frequent vertigo, headache, neck stiffness and transient nausea. She is taking numerous medications for hypertension and Raynaud's phenomenon. Her history includes several rear end collisions and numerous falls over the past ten years. A retired nurse, she had had numerous episodes of low back pain after lifting patients. Examination overall is unremarkable except for marked limitation of the lower cervical spine during motion palpation. No paresthesias are reported, and the pinwheel examination is noncontributory. Laboratory tests indicate marginal anemia with a slight decrease in the hematocrit. Blood pressure, pulse and rhythm are stable.

Review indicates rather extensive degenerative discogenic spondylosis. Small osteophytic spur formations are noted throughout the contiguous body plate margins from C3 through C7. Those located at the posterior margins may be causing foraminal intrusion but, without commensurate paresthesia or evidence of nerve root involvement, are considered quiescent at this time. The covertebral joints of Luschka demonstrate with arthrosis, including oblique extension of proliferation between C5 and C6 and C6 and C7. Vertebral artery compromise is problematical.

Where is the greatest degree of head and/or neck motion occurring? Are hypomobility and fixation present? What other findings are of interest and concern, and do these affect your treatment procedure?

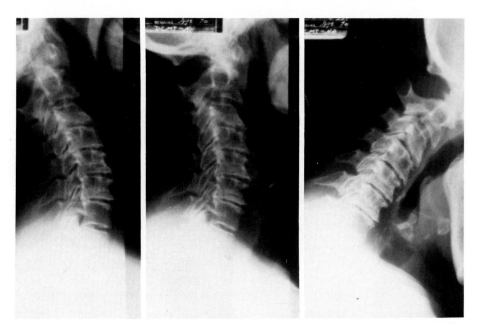

Fig. 2.6C. Ida S.

Examination of the three views in Fig. 2.6C reveals marked hypomobility and fixation from C3 through C7. Nearly all motion of the head and neck occurs above C3. A tendency towards forward displacement of the head and neck above C3 is noted. This lack of "motoricity" is due to ligamentous fixation associated with discal degeneration. The posterior zygapophyseal articulations have generally been spared, and thus lateral rotation and moderate segmental motion are maintained, albeit limited. This lack of facet involvement also explains the minimal pain expression. You will note the small radiolucent streaking within the intervertebral discs between C3 and C4 and C4 and C5 in the flexion view, indicative of the vacuum phenomenon, a pathognomonic sign of discal degeneration.

By now you should have also wondered about the posterior arch of C1. The anterior tubercle is well visualized. Platybasia or basilar impression is not suspect. The protrusion extending downward from the base of the skull represents the posterior lip of the foramen magnum. This represents *agenesis of the posterior arch of C1.* Should your manipulative techniques call for posterior arch contacts, you will be forced to modify! This form of variation rarely produces neurological complication. The lack of basilar impression would suggest that the articular facets of the atlantooccipital articulation are intact, and as described above, motoricity at this level is maintained.

Case 2.7

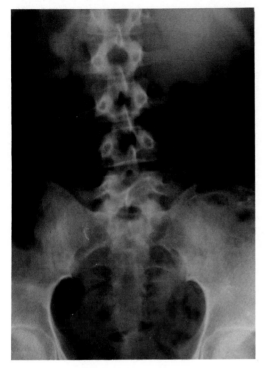

Fig. 2.7A.   Kathy P.

This 18-year-old woman was radiographed as part of a preemployment examination. She was seeking employment as a nurse's aide which requires frequent heavy lifting and much bending.

Kathy denies any previous back trouble or complaint. No serious illness or surgery has been reported. The physical examination suggests a minimal lumbar scoliosis with concavity on the right. Orthopedic and neurological testing are noncontributory.

After review of the film (Fig. 2.7A), you should note a rather blatant defect. What biomechanical factors must be considered? In answering this question, use some imagination. Is Kathy restricted in any movements? Can these variations of mobility predispose to later change? Are these expected to change significantly with certain activities, and lastly do you think that any particular type of treatment is indicated?

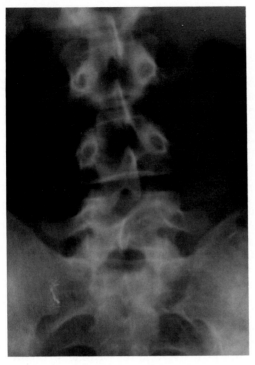

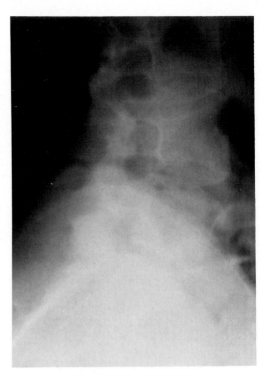

Fig. 2.7B. Kathy P.

Fig. 2.7C. Kathy P.

Total *agenesis* of the inferior articular process and the inferior one half of the lamina of L4 is seen on the right (Fig. 2.7B). This represents a total lack of support to the posterior motor unit of L4 on one side. Note how the L5 laminae, arch, and superior articular process on the right suggest compensatory architectural asymmetry, in an attempt to stabilize.

This agenesis represents loss of the L4–L5 anchoring mechanism on the right. As in unilateral spondylolysis, this lack of rotational constraint on one side will allow abnormal torsion and rotational stress (Fig. 2.7C) to the intervertebral disc, contralateral facets and neural arch (26). Accelerated and excessive fibrillation of the disc will occur, predisposing to degenerative breakdown. Possible stress or fatigue frac-

ture to the opposite neural arch and possible facet arthrosis might well be sequelae. These changes will occur over a long period of time.

Of more concern now is that the "gap" is filled with thick, dense fibrocartilaginous tissue. While sufficient to provide some degree of positional stability, it will not withstand the typical stress of an articular process, nor will it provide the usual fortification against protrusion by the disc. This is a very unstable motor unit. Kathy must be extremely cautious with heavy lifting, right lateral bending, and hyperextension of the low back. Fortunately she has bilateral sagittal facet facings between L5 and S1 to help provide some stability. Unless symptom expression dictates, treatment is not indicated.

Case 2.8

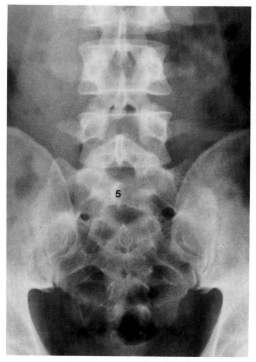

Fig. 2.8A. Howard N.

Howard is a 34-year-old man who works in the heating and air conditioning business as an installer and mechanic. His work is often heavy and awkward.

Howard reports that he has had numerous low back aches over the past few years but that recently these have become much worse. Now sharp pain is experienced in the middle low back. No radiation or paresthesias are reported.

Antalgic posture is noted, with difficulty in getting up from a seated position. No definite right or left leaning is seen. Rest has helped but only temporarily.

Historically, Howard has never had any serious illness or accidents and has had no surgery, except for a tonsillectomy at age six. Examination elicits sharp point tenderness near midline at the level of L3–L4 and L4–L5. Bilateral paraspinal muscular splinting is seen. Deep tendon re-

flexes and neurological evaluation are normal. Laboratory tests are not called for. The patient is overweight by 25 pounds, carrying about 20 of these as a pendulous abdomen. He's not a beer drinker—just loves to eat!

The acute episode of pain began after three days of installing overhead duct work. He noticed the discomfort progressively worsening and on the advice of his family physician began sleeping on a heating pad. This morning he could hardly get out of bed. Once up, the antalgic posture forced him to stoop forward in a central position, but with time and effort he was able to stand upright without sharp pain.

What is your clinical hunch at this point? An acute disc? Are there any findings on the AP radiograph (Fig. 2.8A) which would suggest a biomechanical basis for Howard's problem?

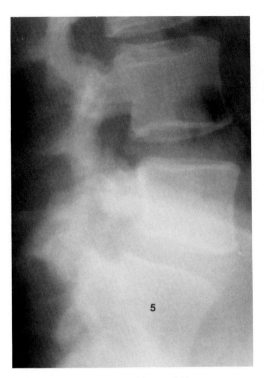

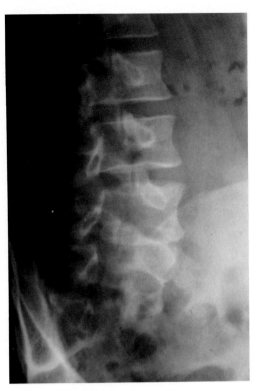

Fig. 2.8B. Howard N.

Fig. 2.8C. Howard N.

Careful review of the AP film indicates bilateral absence of the laminae of L4. No surgery has ever been done. While the appearance is similar to a bilateral surgical laminectomy (rarely performed), it is in fact the result of agenesis—an *autolaminectomy*. As might be anticipated with agenesis of the laminae, the anchoring mechanism is lost between the anterior and posterior motor unit. A grade 1 *spondylolisthesis* of L4 on L5 is seen (Fig. 2.8B). The bilateral spondylolysis of the pars in this case is moot due to the agenesis of the pars and laminae (Fig. 2.8C). In addition, the AP view presents with complete *sacralization* of L5 (24). The inferior articular processes of L5 are bilaterally underdeveloped. (No evidence of neoarthrosis is seen.) Note the bilateral fusion of the transverse processes with the sacral alae.

Howard's complaint is due to soft-tissue insult and/or injury, the result of "pincher effect" by the articular processes above and below the area of agenesis, following three days of overhead work with hyperextension of the lumbar spine. The resultant soft-tissue swelling was exacerbated by the use of heat. It is well to remember that with soft-tissue irritation the employment of ice or cryotherapy is recommended in the acute phase.

While an acute lumbar disc syndrome was possible, based on the presenting complaint, the lack of lateral antalgic posture and neuropathy would have indicated a central prolapse and/or protrusion. This type of disc lesion is unusual and would have presented with little, if any, positional relief when weight bearing.

Howard's response to treatment was prompt. He now avoids hyperextension of the lumbar spine and employs an orthopedic support while engaging in heavy work.

Case 2.9

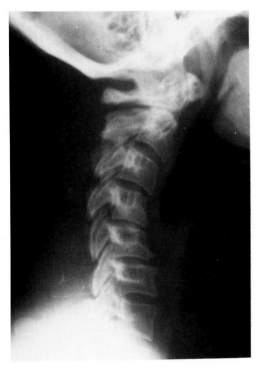

Fig. 2.9A. Triscia J.

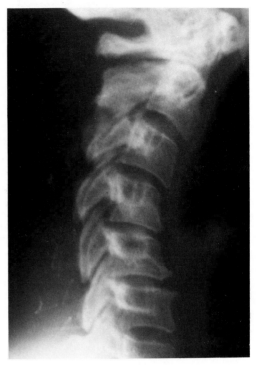

Fig. 2.9B. Triscia J.

Triscia's films (Fig. 2.9, *A* and *B*) are provided merely to include a case of multilevel surgical laminectomy. This 34-year-old woman was involved in a major auto accident five years ago. Severe head and neck injuries were sustained with resultant laminae fractures and attending meningeal swelling. A *surgical laminectomy* was done, removing the spinous processes as well, from C2 to C6. This procedure not only allowed for cleaning up of the fracture debris but allowed for decompression of the meningeal components. Recovery was satisfactory with no paralysis.

As you can see from these films, Triscia

has a marked reversal of the cervical lordosis. This is the result of marked soft-tissue and ligamentous tearing with the formation of cicatricial fixation. In addition, an early cervical degenerative discogenic spondylosis is seen between C4 and C5 and C5 and C6.

With periodic cervical manipulation with gentle rotary movements, the patient gets along very well. Only time will tell to what extent discal degeneration and the accelerated aging process will develop as sequelae of this accident. Incidentally, the fine radiopaque lines in the posterior soft tissue at C5–C6 are residual surgical sutures of no clinical importance at this time.

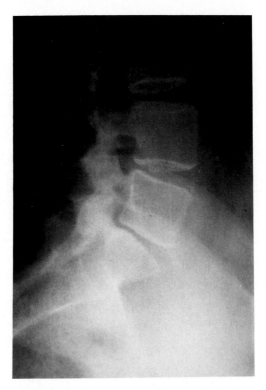

Fig. 2.10. Hypoplastic intervertebral disc.

The decreased height of the L5-S1 intervertebral disc is well seen in Fig. 2.10. Lacking the antalgic rigidity of an acute disc prolapse or protrusion, the discal thinning would generally be considered the result of degeneration.

With discal degeneration, referred to as degenerative disc disease, marginal thickening, sclerosis and, frequently, osteophytic spur formation would be anticipated of the contiguous body plate margins. In this case, none of these findings are noted. Examination indicates clearly defined body plate margins. While decreased interosseous spacing and foraminal alteration are seen, the remaining criterion of discal degeneration or arthrosis is lacking. Thus, by differential exclusion the presence of a *hypoplastic or underdeveloped disc* is concluded.

Now a note of caution. It is relatively impossible to differentiate a hypoplastic disc from an early discal degeneration prior to marginal changes. The age of the patient is helpful—over 40—and serial films taken at six-month intervals are normally conclusive. We have seen some refer to discal degeneration in patients under 20. This is unlikely except when it is traumatically or pathologically induced. The intervertebral disc does not normally complete its growth until after age 16 (27). It is therefore unrealistic to propose degeneration prior to cessation of growth, with the exceptions previously noted.

Hypoplastic discs, although developmental in origin, are nonetheless responsible for altered biomechanics similar to those produced via discal degeneration.

Case 2.10

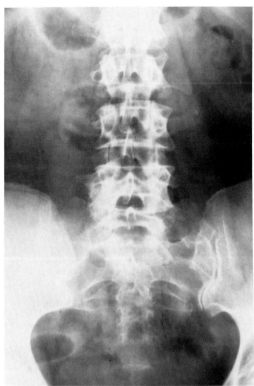

Fig. 2.11A. Elmer P.

Is bilateral sacralization usually associated with facet irritation?

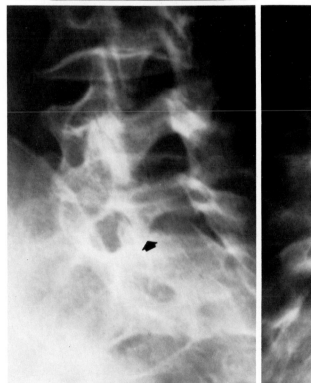

Fig. 2.11B. Elmer P.

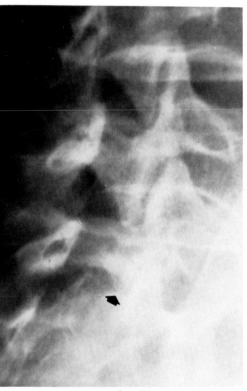

Fig. 2.11C. Elmer P.

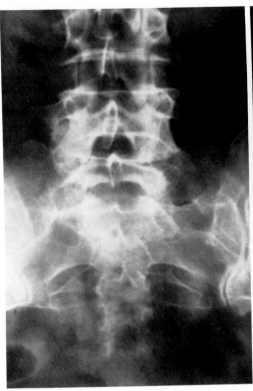

Fig. 2.11D. Elmer P.

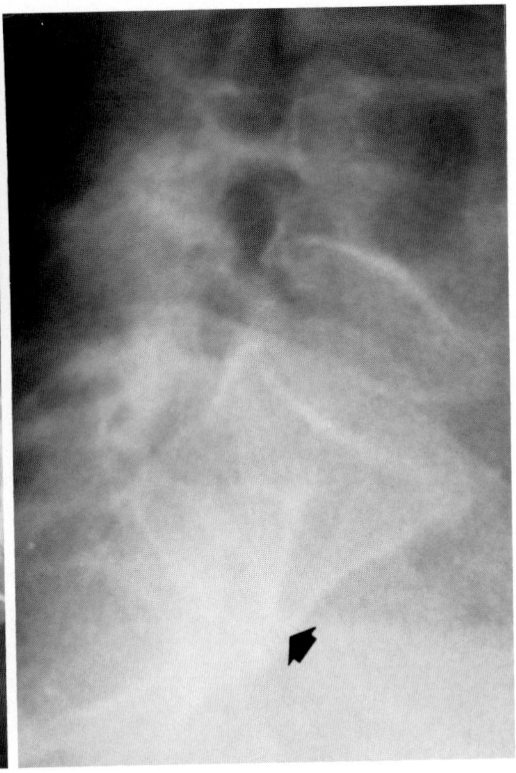

Fig. 2.11E. Elmer P.

Sacralization, or the tendency towards fusion between the L5 segment and the sacrum, is a frequent anatomical variation encountered in the low back (24).

In most cases the anatomical variation demonstrates with large spatulated transverse processes of L5 which fuse with the sacral alae. This anomalous formation is typically found in cases with an associated underdevelopment in the length of the L5 inferior articular processes. It appears to be Mother Nature's way of compensation and adaptation to ensure a balanced posture. In addition, this variation is usually associated with a rudimentary lumbosacral disc, *arrow* in Fig. 2.11E.

In Fig. 2.11, you will note that in *A* and *D* the large transverse processes of L5 have joined with the sacral alae. The lack of reactive sclerosis at the site of fusion indicates that complete fusion has occurred and that no neoarthrosis has developed. In *B* and *C* of Fig. 2.11, the anatomical deficiency in the length of the L5 inferior articular processes and facets is well demonstrated.

As we shall see, the variation of facets, i.e., asymmetry, is a frequent finding, and only when compensation fails to occur does it generally produce clinical or biomechanical variations of importance.

Case 2.11

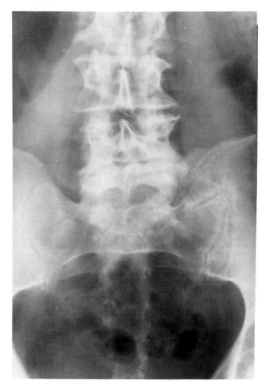

Fig. 2.12A. Dave L.

A 56-year-old carpenter, Dave has had low back pain off and on again for years. Usually the pain is dull and progressively worsens throughout the day. Rest helps but brings only temporary relief.

History reveals that many years ago he was forced to take six weeks off work due to severe left sciatic pain. While rest and conservative manipulative management were successful in returning him to work, he has had periodic episodes of similar pain following excessive or heavy work.

Last week, Dave developed a severe, sharp pain in the right L-S area which extended outward into the buttock. It was a different type of pain than was usual, being sharp and stab-like, which has not eased much with rest or heat.

Your examination does not uncover any positive, objective neurological or or-thopedic findings. Mild paraspinal tenderness with spasm is found in the right lumbar and lumbosacral region. Point tenderness and pain are found over the right superior sacroiliac articulation and seems to radiate outward into the soft tissue of the buttock. While it is difficult for Dave to get up from a sitting position, once up he is able to stand erect with only minimal antalgic leaning. No paresthesias are noted.

From the radiograph (Fig. 2.12A) you can explain the history of chronicity, make a reasonable assumption concerning the previous acute episode with sciatic involvement, and explain not only how the present condition developed but what probable condition is responsible for his current pain—can't you?

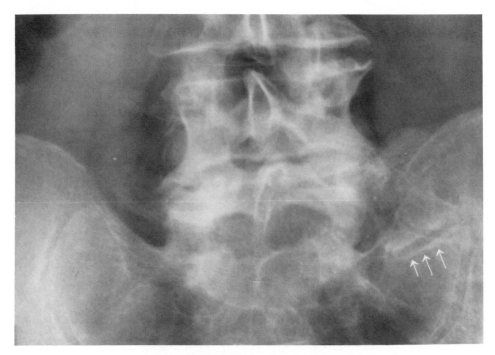

Fig. 2.12B. Dave L.

Review of Fig. 2.12 indicates that Dave has had frequent insults to his low back. The numerous osteophytes suggest a prior local periosteitis, presumably of discal origin. The left lateral flexion subluxation of L4 on L5 is marked, and the decreased intervertebral disc height obvious. Coupled with the history, these findings indicate a probable prior acute lumbar disc syndrome, i.e., prolapse or protrusion, at L4-L5 on the left. The remaining lumbar spondylosis is due to altered weight bearing, the result of the disc lesion, coupled with the architectural changes of L5-S1 on the right.

You will note, at the *arrows* on the right (Fig. 2.12B), a large spatulated transverse process of L5 which has developed a *neoarthrosis* with the sacral ala. Fre-quently this *new joint* seems to be associated with an anatomical deficiency in the length of the inferior articular process of L5 on the ipsilateral side. It appears as Mother Nature's way of balancing the lumbosacral complex.

With the new joint formation comes the development of an attending synovium or lubricating sac which, like all synovium, is subject to insult and/or injury. The marginal sclerosis and thickening seen in Fig. 2.12B indicates that chronic, repetitive synovitis has occurred with resultant marginal arthrosis of this neoarthrosis (20). With acute exacerbation of this chronic synovial insult comes the localized pain as described by Dave. The absence of nerve root involvement is a significant differential finding.

Case 2.12

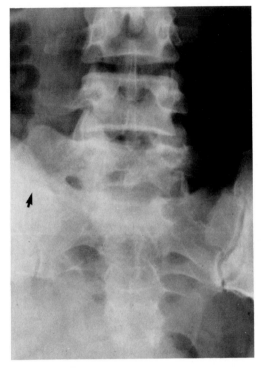

Fig. 2.13A.   Dana W.

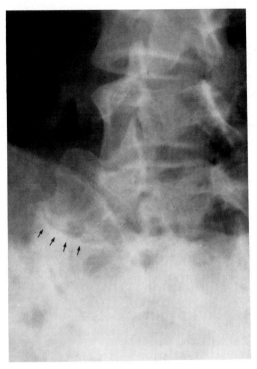

Fig. 2.13B.   Dana W.

By this time you should be quite familiar with a *neoarthrosis formation* between a large spatulated transverse process and the sacral ala. It is not uncommon. As mentioned, it seems precipitated by an anatomical deficiency in the length of the L5 inferior articular process. Dana's case "fits." The *small arrows* in Fig. 2.13B indicate marked thickening and sclerosis, a sign of chronicity and commensurate with arthrosis. Probable chronic recurrent synovial insult or irritation would be suspect and did occur from time to time with stress and activity.

Dana is a 37-year-old postal worker and outdoor enthusiast. As he walks most of his route everyday, we instructed him to carry his bag on his right shoulder to lessen the stress to the left L-S area. He refused, insisting that being right handed would make it impossible. Also, while we did not offer restriction on his hunting or fishing, we did ask that he be careful while snowmobiling to avoid any unnecessary jolts by sticking to the prepared trails. He just smiled.

Soon after the Christmas holidays and the usual overtime workload, Dana planned a winter vacation to enjoy our beautiful snow-covered ski and snowmobile trails.

His lower back had been quite sore with an occasional twinge of pain. He considered it a transient irritation caused by overwork and fatigue. On his first day of vacation his robust personality was accentuated by alcohol. While forging new trails on his snowmobile, his machine unexpectedly hit a ditch throwing Dana's upper torso severely to the left, while at the same time experiencing a severe concussion of forces to his low back. His vacation ended. The next morning he presented for examination, and films (Fig. 2.13C and D) were reviewed.

A radiolucent fracture cleft is seen (Fig. 2.13D, *arrow*) running obliquely from superior to inferior of the L5 transverse process. The fracture margins are relatively smooth—unusual for a fresh traumatic fracture. The lack of reactive sclerosis or callus formation confirms its recent vintage. With the recent history in this case it is more appropriately a *stress* or *fatigue fracture*. Retrospectively, we are more convinced in that healing took nearly three months—far longer than would be anticipated in a pure traumatic fracture. You will note that good apposition of the fracture fragment was maintained.

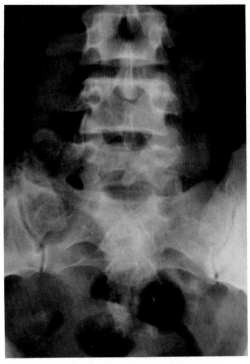

Fig. 2.13C.   Dana W.

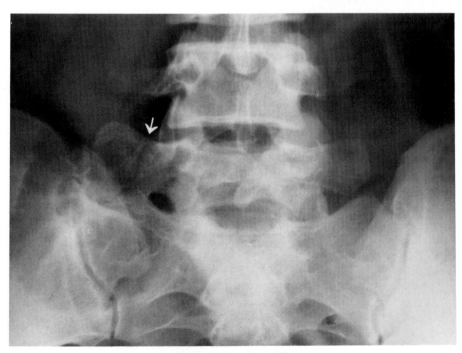

Fig. 2.13D.   Dana W.

Case 2.13

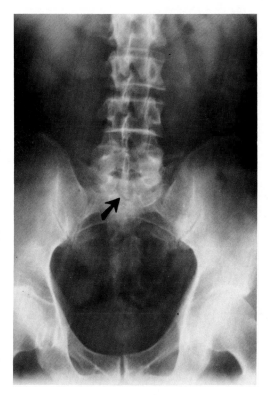

Fig. 2.14A. Garvin F.

Garvin is a 62-year-old Caucasian man who presented for examination and treatment for acute, sharp pain located near midline at the lumbosacral complex. Localized erythema was noted, as well as point tenderness. No neuropathy or paresthesias were encountered. Lasegue's, Braggard's and stiff-leg-raising tests were all moderately positive, bilaterally.

The patient had been painting and redecorating his home over the past two weeks of his vacation. After repairing and painting the eaves trough yesterday, he began experiencing pain which has progressively worsened.

In his attempt to gain relief, the patient slept on a heating pad all night. This morning he had a very difficult time in getting out of bed.

This condition (Fig. 2.14A, *arrow*) was initially described as a clinical entity by Earl A. Rich, D.C., in the early 1950s. It is a frequent finding and not always symptomatic. The lateral radiograph in this condition is noncontributory. Is the condition congenital, posttraumatic or pathological?

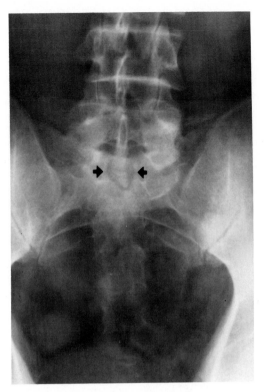

Fig. 2.14B.   Garvin F.

You will note that a spina bifida occulta is present due to failure in closure of the S1 neural arch. In addition, an elongated spinous process of L5 is seen. This combination of findings is characteristic of the "*knife clasp*" syndrome (Fig. 2.14, *A* and *B*).

During hyperextension of the lumbosacral complex, as in working overhead on an eaves trough while standing on a ladder, a soft-tissue compression is produced by a tendency towards invagination by the spinous process into the sacral fault.

This compression causes insult and/or injury with resultant soft-tissue irritation, swelling and pain. It rarely produces neural involvement.

In this case, close inspection suggests that Garvin also has a separation of the distal end of the L5 spinous process, i.e., a persistent apophysis. This latter finding is coincidental and is not typical of the "knife clasp" syndrome.

As this condition is congenital in origin, control of those activities which predispose towards symptom expression is the treatment of choice, i.e., prevention. When acute exacerbation does occur, the symptom picture is one relating to soft-tissue insult with swelling and/or edema. Therefore, the use of heat is contraindicated in the initial phase. Cryotherapy or ice packs is recommended for dissipation of the symptom producing soft-tissue swelling.

Case 2.14

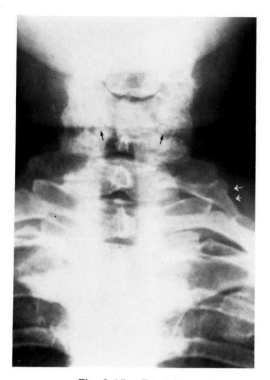

Fig. 2.15.   Ethel A.

Ethel (Fig. 2.15) is a 54-year-old Caucasian woman who reports with transient vertigo and marked stiffness with aching of the neck upon arising in the morning. This complaint is of long standing. Recently, after refurbishing a new home, she developed pain and fleeting numbness in the right shoulder, arm and hand.

As noted by the *black arrows* in Fig. 2.15, this patient has bilateral covertebral joints of Luschka arthrosis between C5 and C6. Slight obliquity of the proliferative osteophytic formation is noted on the left. This alteration explains transient vertigo should the position of the head and neck allow transient compression of the vertebral artery with diminished blood flow.

Her stiffness and ache in the morning is due to the decreased interosseous spacing subluxation between C5 and C6 and the moderate posterior vertebral joint arthrosis noted throughout the lower cervical spine.

After Ethel moved to her new house, she excitedly began hanging new heavy draperies. She spent days hanging, changing, pinning—all with her arms elevated. She was unaware that a *cervical rib* (*white arrows*) was present. The repetitive nature of her experience produced a compression irritation to the scalenus muscle and its contiguous neurovascular structures, resulting in the symptom expression of transient shoulder, arm and hand paresthesias.

Case 2.15

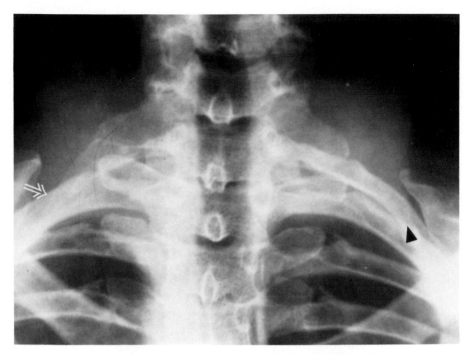

Fig. 2.16. Henry D.

Henry D. (Fig. 2.16) is a very busy dry wall contractor. Since getting into business for himself about one year ago, he has experienced frequent periods of numbness and tingling of both hands, particularly on the left.

Since becoming his own boss, Henry has been working a little harder and spending more hours on the job. The rash of new business also included much ceiling work. Unlike Ethel A. above, Henry had had transient attacks of paresthesias before, but with a day or two of rest, it would ease, and he would forget about it. Now he has been at it almost constantly and has pushed it to a near chronic state.

The *double white arrow* on the left in Fig. 2.16 is a typical *cervical rib*, demonstrating with the rudimentary rib head with tapering extension angled somewhat downward. The *black arrowhead* indicates a more developed, albeit still anomalous, C7 rib on the right. This bilateral involvement is unusual but does occur.

Case 2.16

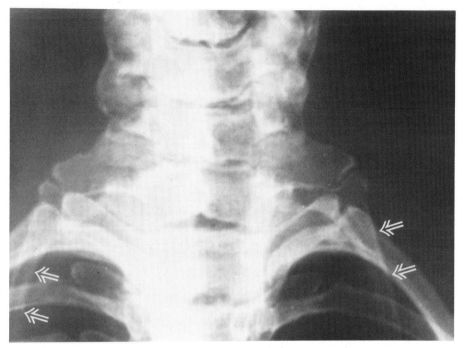

Fig. 2.17. John D.

With the last two cases, plus that of John D. (Fig. 2.17), you are now probably an expert at picking up cervical ribs on an x-ray. This case, as indicated by the bilateral *double arrows*, presents with the typical appearance of the *bilateral cervical rib syndrome*. It may of course be unilateral or bilateral, and the clinical picture is usually associated with the side(s) of involvement.

Now a word of *caution*. Often, elongation or overdevelopment in the length of the transverse process at C7 can induce irritation and symptoms similar to the cervical rib syndrome. In this instance, however, you must categorize and refer to it as a scalenus anticus syndrome and NOT as a cervical rib syndrome.

Only after demonstration of a rudimentary rib head, regardless of size, and an articulation between it and the transverse process can you technically term it a cervical rib.

It is well to remember also that the cervical rib is usually attended by cartilaginous extension from its distal end, which at times reaches far anterior seeking attachment (23). This formation is rarely visible on your film but can certainly complicate the clinical course in what might otherwise be considered a simple anatomical variant.

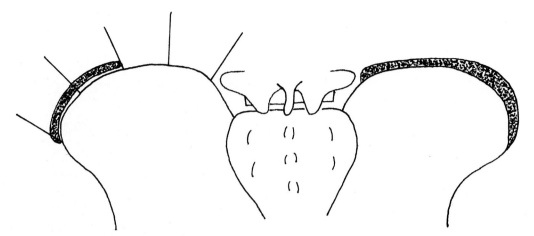

Fig. 2.18. Schematic of Risser's sign. Ossification of the iliac crests as an indicator of skeletal maturation. The iliac epiphysis begins its ossification at the anterior iliac crest and progresses posteriorly. The iliac crest is divided into four quarters, and the degree of maturation is designated as the amount of progression. On the left above is noted epiphyseal growth of nearly half of the crest, thus the Risser's sign is 2+. On the right, complete epiphyseal appearance and ossification have occurred—a Risser's 5+ sign (21).

A definite correlation with complete fusion of the iliac epiphysis and cessation of skeletal growth in height has been shown. This measurement is particularly important when designing an appropriate therapeutic regime in scoliosis and other disorders of children and adolescents. The iliac epiphysis begins ossification at the anterior crest and gradually progresses posteriorly. It may occasionally do so in a staggered or fragmented manner, normally. Once complete ossification of the epiphysis occurs, fusion with the ilium takes place. *Measurement of this epiphyseal ossification* was first described by Risser. The iliac crest is divided into four quarters, designating the degree of excursion as 1+ with 25 percent completed, 2+ with 50 percent completed, 3+ with 75 percent completed, 4+ for complete excursion prior to fusion, and 5+ when excursion and fusion to the ilium are complete. The iliac epiphysis appears at puberty (21).

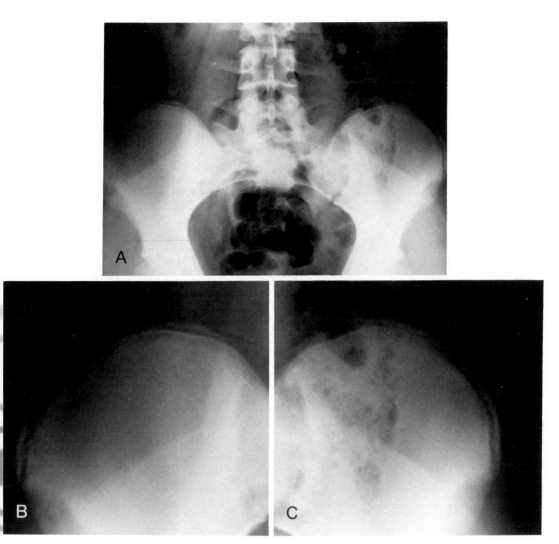

Fig. 2.19. *A*: Late adolescent pelvis as measured by Risser's sign. *B*: Close up of left iliac crest in *A*. Notice no attempt as yet of the epiphysis to fuse, indicating incomplete ossification. *C*: Close up of right iliac crest in *A*. The staggered or fragmented ossification of the epiphysis is normal.

Case 2.17

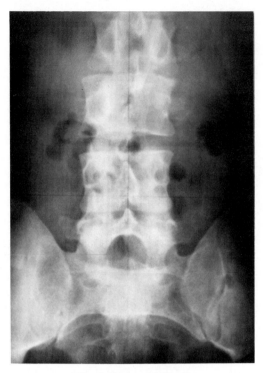

Fig. 2.20A. Phillip T.

Phillip is a 28-year-old man who presented with marked paraspinal muscle splinting and tenderness from the L4 through the S1 region on the left. No paresthesias are noted.

He reports that on the previous day he had loaded his snow blower onto a truck and, while doing so, his left foot slipped on ice, causing a sudden, severe strain to his low back. Pain has been constant since, even though he immediately put a heating pad on the injured area and stayed off his feet until this morning.

Two diagnostic and radiographic questions arise. First, what is the source of Phillip's pain, and do you have any suggestions regarding appropriate treatment? Next, is there any other radiographic finding of significance, and if so, what condition must be ruled out?

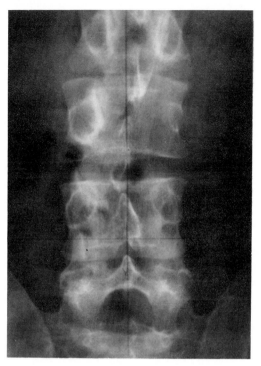

Fig. 2.20B. Phillip T.

A moderately severe left *lateral flexion subluxation* of L4 on L5 is seen with attending interarticular facet imbrication (Fig. 2.20, *A* and *B*). Disruption of Hadley's "S" line can also be seen. Probable interarticular facet synovitis and/or irritation are suspect. The patient's employment of heat following an acute injury of this type, while perhaps soothing the muscular strain, also facilitated the developing synovitis due to increased vascularity. Cryotherapy or ice packs is more efficacious in helping to reduce swelling and therefore pain. It is well to ask your patient "when was the last time you saw a heating pad used on a football field?" Cryotherapy and manipulation were employed with uneventful recovery.

Careful review of the films also reveals a *"one-eyed pedicle"* of L3. In this case a rudimentary pedicle on the right is noted (Fig. 2.20C). When coupled with the patient's age and lack of significant clinical illness, an *anomalous development* is probable. Tomography was utilized for verification.

The one-eyed pedicle or one-eyed vertebra sign is an important differential point between osteolytic metastasis and multiple myeloma. While this sign develops relatively early in some osteolytic metastasis, the lack of red bone marrow in the pedicle rarely causes involvement by multiple myeloma (12, 23).

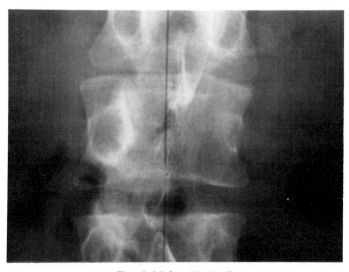

Fig. 2.20C. Phillip T.

Case 2.18

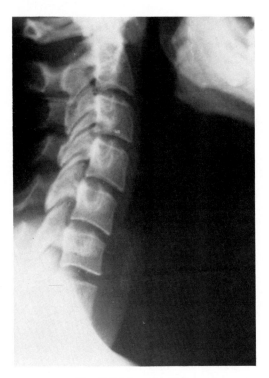

Fig. 2.21A. David B.

David is a 39-year-old postal worker who has noticed a decrease of energy and increased overall aching of head, neck and upper thoracic region for the past three to four months. He reports transient nausea, vertigo, lethargy and fleeting periods of low-grade fever.

At examination a marked flattening of the cervical and thoracic curves is noted without palpable tenderness. All laboratory tests are within the outer limits of normal, although the WBC was slightly elevated on a recheck.

Radiographs A and B in Fig. 2.21 were selected for your review due to the rather obvious, but often overlooked, problem which led to the correct disposition of this case.

As with all diagnoses, try to correlate clinical complaints with objective findings. Your system or pattern of radiographic review will help you to avoid many pitfalls.

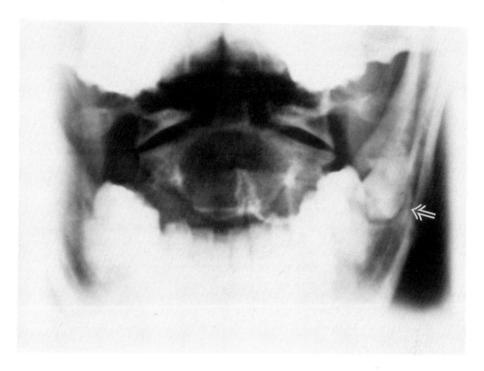

Fig. 2.21*B.*   David B.

As indicated by the *arrow* in Fig. 2.21B, this patient has an unerupted, or more accurately in this instance, an impaction of his third molar on the right—his *wisdom tooth.* Retrospective review of the lateral will just barely allow your observation of it. Notice the halo of radiolucency surrounding nearly two thirds of the tooth. This finding is highly suggestive of abscess or the collection of suppurative material around the tooth (23). This explains the clinical picture of low-grade infection. The patient was referred to his dentist, and after a short course of antibiotic therapy the tooth was extracted. An uneventful recovery followed.

This case is included for two specific reasons. First, to point out the necessity of adequately defining all structures on your films, and second, to remind you that correlation of clinical and radiographic findings cannot be overemphasized. This last point is significant in that not all impacted wisdom teeth are of clinical importance at the time of their discovery. Many are found incidentally and, if acted upon at that time, might well save the patient unnecessary suffering at some future date.

Section 3

Biomechanical Considerations

Case 3.1

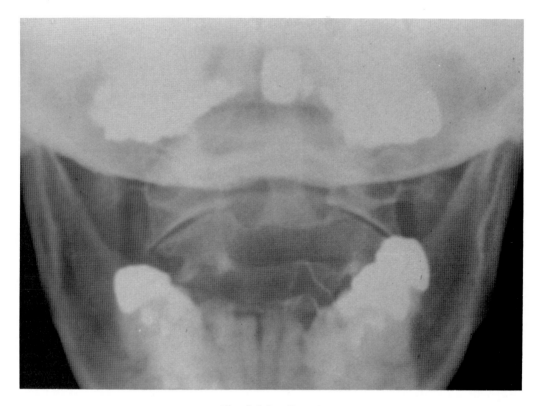

Fig. 3.1 A. Rose L.

While at work this morning, Rose had a severe headache, transient nausea and unexplained stiffness of her neck. No trauma was reported, but she admitted to having the habit of cradling the telephone between her head and left shoulder while at work as a busy receptionist. Recently she had been even busier than usual, work-ing overtime. This history coupled with a habit of falling asleep while watching TV and lying on the couch clinched the etiol-ogy.

Remember Chiropractic 101? Then you will be able to identify the significance of *arrows A* and *B* in Fig. 3.1B.

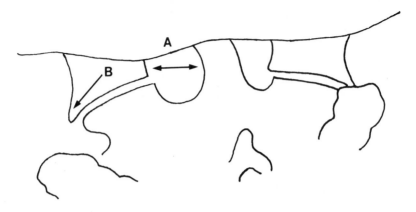

Fig. 3.1B. Schematic of Fig. 3.1A.

While slight off-centering is noted of the odontoid process due to minor rotation of C2, its appearance in this case is basically the result of developmental origin. A "bent" odontoid—not an unusual finding.

Arrow A represents the *lateral* atlanto-dental interval (ADI). This interspace, between the odontoid and lateral masses of C2, varies with rotation and/or lateral mobility of one segment in relationship to the other. The *lateral* ADI is markedly increased on the left. This when coupled with the left lateral movement of C1 on C2, *arrow B*, would indicate *levorotatory subluxation of C1 on C2.*

This biomechanical disrelationship between C1 and C2 was due to repetitive postural stress, ligamentous fatigue and diminution of muscular tonicity. The attending symptom complex was essentially the result of spasm of the suboccipital triangle and its neurovascular components.

It is well to point out that while variations of the lateral ADI are typically the result of altered biomechanics, alterations of the *anterior* ADI are usually due to changes within the synovium lying just posterior to the anterior tubercle of C1, e.g., rheumatoid arthritis (1, 18, 19).

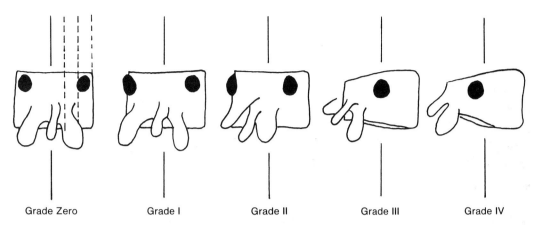

| Grade Zero | Grade I | Grade II | Grade III | Grade IV |

Fig. 3.2. Vertebral rotation. The distance between the pedicle and the vertebral margin is measured. As the vertebra rotates, the pedicle approaches midline, passing it in grade IV, with the pedicle-vertebral margin increasing. (Adapted from Nash and Moe.)

The *measurement of vertebral rotation* has been of importance to the chiropractor since the advent of spinography. Many systems have been and are utilized. A problem with many systems has been the selection of a point of reference. The use of spinous processes, laminae junction, vertebral margins, etc., has been less than dependable due to the numerous anatomical variations which occur at these sites. While the system shown in Fig. 3.2 was originally designed to measure the degree of rotation to the apical vertebra in sco-liosis, its practical application in spinography is apparent. The system measures the pedicle displacement from the vertebral margin. By dividing each half of the vertebral body into thirds and determining the pedicle location in reference to each sector, as it nears midline, gradings of 0, I, II, III and IV are possible. Grade 0 is normal with equidistance between the pedicle and vertebral margins on either side. Grade IV demonstrates the pedicle beyond midline (17, 21).

Case 3.2

Case 3.3

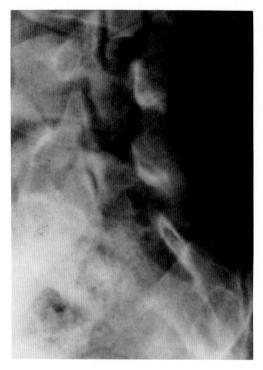

Fig. 3.3. Darryl J.

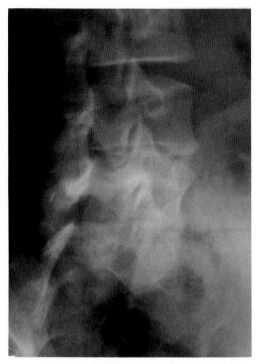

Fig. 3.4. Lance P.

These two gentlemen, and their oblique radiographs, were selected as typical examples of *interarticular facet imbrication*, i.e., subluxation. Both involve the L5-S1 level. In Darryl's case (Fig. 3.3), the lesion is noted on his left (seen in the RAO projection), and in Lance's (Fig. 3.4), on the right (seen in the LAO projection). You will note the telescoping or jamming of the superior articular facet of S1 ("Scotty dog's ear") into the underside of the pars interarticularis of L5. Attending alteration of

the L5-S1 interarticular facet interspace is well demonstrated. Probable interarticular facet synovitis would be anticipated.

Additionally, you will note that a dense sclerotic thickening is occurring of the pars near its inferior margin. This sclerotic alteration is probable evidence of chronic, repetitive stress. Unless correction or adaptation of the imbrication is made, the progression of this sclerotic alteration into posterior vertebral joint arthrosis is probable in time.

Case 3.4

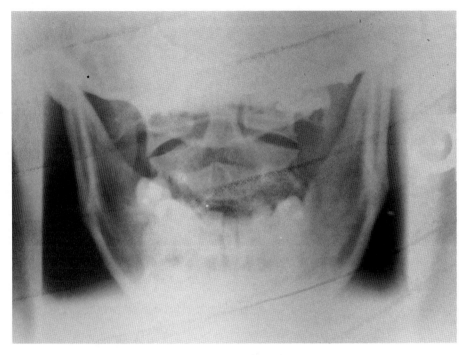

Fig. 3.5A.   Leslie W.

Of importance to most chiropractors is the biomechanical relationship of the atlantooccipital and atlantoaxial segments. The numerous physiological and pathophysiological responses produced by alterations at these levels are legendary. Altered function revolves around neurovascular involvement but also includes kinetic and postural stresses. These effects are both locally and peripherally expressed, dependent on the type of involvement.

While numerous variations are possible in positional disrelationships, the sagittal, coronal and transverse plane movements govern nearly all altered states. Without fracture, all abnormal motions involve at least two of the three planes of movement. It must be born in mind that with lateral deviation of one segment in relation to the one above or below (coronal plane), the plane of articulation of the interarticular facets produces involvement in the transverse plane, creating lateral flexion (15). When observing subluxation, one must consider which planes are involved, particularly when establishing corrective therapy.

Leslie W. has a left lateral subluxation of C1 on C2, as seen in Fig. 3.5. In addition, due to the plane of articulation, an attending left lateral flexion is also noted. This combination is often referred to as a *levorotatory subluxation*.

When seen in the absence of fracture or architectural anomaly, this finding may well produce symptom expression both locally and peripherally. What produces these symptoms *in addition to* neurovascular, kinetic and postural stress?

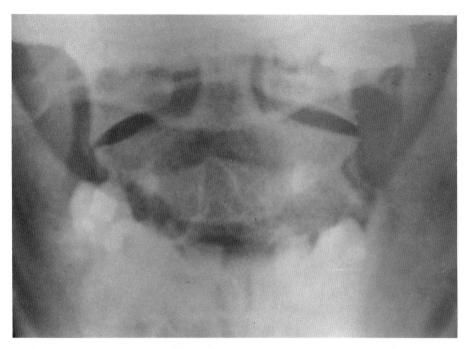

Fig. 3.5*B*.   Leslie W.

In any alteration involving the biomechanical relationships of amphiarthrodial or diarthrodial joints, the capsule and synovial membranes are of great importance. Their integrity and degree of homeostasis determine in large measure the amount of local symptom expression and functional involvement. This occurs by accentuation of both the kinetic and proprioceptive response.

In Leslie's case (Fig. 3.5*B*), mechanical stress to the interarticular synovium at both the lateral masses and that located between the odontoid process and anterior tubercle of C1 is likely. Increased tension of the capsular membrane is also encountered. As a result, altered biomechanical rhythm and function are produced.

Significant factors which contribute to your correct radiographic evaluation of subluxation include the recognition of ligamentous involvement, particularly of the transverse and cruciform ligaments when examining C1-C2, and the utilization of the pedicle-lateral vertebral body margin distance in the determination of rotation (below C1). Due to the high incidence of anomalous developmental asymmetry, use of the spinous process or laminae junction as a point of reference is prone to error. At the C1-C2 level, utilization of the lateral atlantodental (odontoid) interspace (ADI) is helpful.

This case and comment are offered to bring awareness that each subluxation is capable of producing variable symptoms, dependent upon the extent and degree of many factors. This explains why some radiographically detected subluxations are of more significance clinically than others. Also, it begins to explain the variation in response to treatment, even though two cases are radiographically similar.

Case 3.5

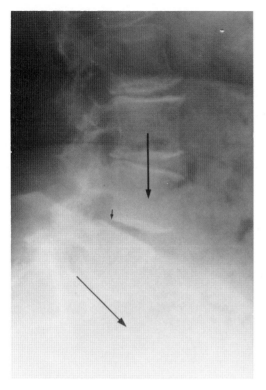

Fig. 3.6A. Yvonne S.

Although Yvonne had hurt her low back by a fall from a horse many years ago, she has had only transient spells of low back pain until recently.

Two months ago she took a job which requires prolonged standing at a bench and a moderate amount of lifting of boxes weighing 25 pounds each.

Her 180 pounds is also a bit of a problem, since she is only 5 foot 3 inches in height.

Her presenting complaint was a dull ache in the low back with fleeting pains into both anterior and anteromedial thighs.

Identify the *arrows* in Fig. 3.6A and their significance. No evidence of spondylolysis was noted on any of the films, including lumbar obliques. Is there evidence of the old injury? Is it of clinical importance at this time? What explanation do you find for the current complaint, and is there a measurement to indicate its severity?

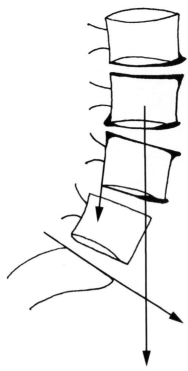

Fig. 3.6*B*.   Yvonne S. Schematic of Fig. 3.6*A*.

Yvonne demonstrates a segmental dis-cogenic spondylosis between L2-L3 and L3-L4. The spur formations, decreased dis-cal height at the posterior one third of each, and their tendency towards hyper-extension suggest an old injury response. This accounts for her chronic, periodic complaint. The posterolateral spur intru-sion at L3-L4 indicates foraminal en-croachment. Neurovascular compromise is problematical.

The sacral base angle, as seen by the *lowermost arrow* in Fig. 3.6, *A* and *B*, is increased, suggesting *anteflexion of the pelvis.*

The forward displacement of Fergus-son's weight-bearing line, the *uppermost arrow* in Fig. 3.6, *A* and *B*, indicates hy-perlordosis of the lumbar spine (15). This combination indicates increased lumbo-sacral instability.

A break of George's line is seen between L4 and L5, the *smaller arrow* in Fig. 3.6, *A* and *B*. The L4 unit demonstrates with an-terolisthesis of L4 on L5. No break or def-icit in the pars interarticularis is demon-strated, however; therefore this is classi-fied as a grade 1 nonspondylolytic spon-dylolisthesis.

The onset of Yvonne's current complaint is the result of insult and/or irritation of the L4-L5 and lumbosacral posterior inter-articular facets due to the stress of work activity combined with the unstable lum-bosacral complex and her overweight con-dition.

Case 3.6

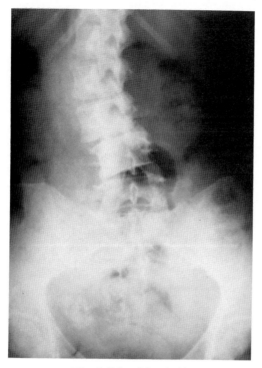

Fig. 3.7A. Marvin H.

Marvin is a 58-year-old man who reports long-standing low back discomfort. Several episodes of sciatic neuropathy and periodic weakness of the left lower extremity have occurred over the past 3 to 4 years. As a young paratrooper, Marvin had had many occasions when he injured his low back, but never seriously enough to require more than bed rest. He has worked in the local bank for the past 30 years as a loan officer.

After a hiking-camping trip with his family three weeks ago (his first ever), constant pain developed in the left L-S region with some moderate extension into the left buttock and posterior thigh. Neu-

rological examination indicates diminished patella reflex on the left. Orthopedic testing produces mild aggravation with stiff leg raising and dorsiflexion of the foot, on the left. All laboratory findings are normal. Mild atrophy of the left leg muscle is noted by measurement.

The film shown in Fig. 3.7A is in the upright or standing view. Is the osteosclerosis of the lumbar spine pathological or physiological in origin? Should Marvin be advised of probable repetitive episodes, or can we assume complete recovery? Can we extrapolate that discal protrusion has occurred? At what level? Is there a term for the type of osteophytic formation seen?

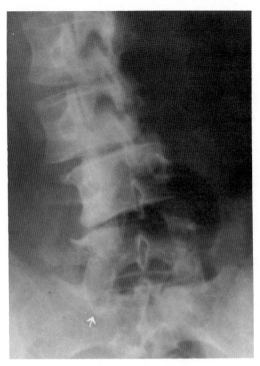

Fig. 3.7*B.*   Marvin H.

Dense sclerotic thickening is noted involving the left lateral one third of the L4 vertebral body. You will note that no evidence of reactive periosteitis, squaring of vertebral end plates, or loss of contiguous architecture by osteolytic destruction is seen. The sclerosis is not "soft" as in condensation. This represents *physiological osteosclerosis* in response to abnormal stress according to Wolff's law; i.e., bone responds dynamically to stresses placed upon it by changing its internal architecture (sclerosis).

Rather marked wedging is noted of the L3-L4 and L4-L5 intervertebral discs. The somewhat concave appearance of the osteophytic spur formation at the left superior margin of L5 suggests a *"traction spur,"* i.e., one which has developed around partially extruded discal material and annular fibers (9).

By extrapolation we can imagine that Marvin has suffered *prolapse* and/or *protrusion* of the *L4-L5 disc*, with the lesion being located lateral to the nerve root on the left. Torsion and discal fibrillation are probable at L3-L4.

No evidence of facet fracture was seen on the other films. Left lateral flexion subluxation of L5 on S1 is noted. This finding is chronic, having produced a *facet-lamina syndrome*, i.e., sclerosis in response to repetitive stress (see the *arrow* in Fig. 3.7*B*). Severe left lateral flexion subluxation with slight levorotatory adaptation of L4 is seen in response to the chronic discal insult. Left *lateral listhesis* of L3 on L4 due to extreme levorotatory adaptation with probable attending ligamentous fibrillation, fixation and possible cicatricial replacement fibrosis of the L3-L4 annular fibers. The overall levorotatory scoliosis of the lumbar spine is seen with concavity on the right. Involvement of the thoracolumbar spine would be anticipated.

Marvin will respond to acute exacerbation due to facet irritation(s) but will be faced with recurrent symptom expression dependent on activity. Manipulation is indicated on a periodic basis to maintain and hopefully regain some interarticular mobility.

Case 3.7

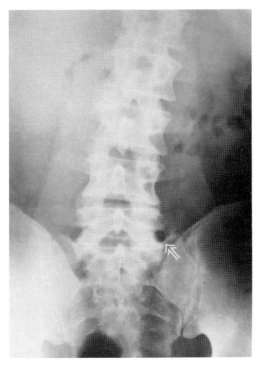

Fig. 3.8A. Andy B.

Andy is a 34-year-old man who is an on-line mechanic at an auto manufacturing firm. He has enjoyed robust health with little back problems until yesterday. After a chain broke on a machine he was hoisting, he quickly tried to grab the load and restrain it. When doing so he felt immediate pain in his low back and down his left leg. Within an hour the pain became so intense that he was barely able to walk and, when doing so, found he had to tilt to the right to relieve the pressure pain in his left leg. He was seen by the company physician, was told he strained the lumbosacral joint, and was instructed to go home for bed rest and application of heat. An aspirin preparation was given for pain.

Andy spent a miserable night with little sound sleep due to the intense pain radiating down the back of the entire left lower extremity into his large toe. The heat felt good but did little to relieve the pain. In the morning the pain was actually worse, and walking was extremely difficult. The left lower extremity felt weak, barely able to support any weight, and all movement was an effort. When he coughed or sneezed the pain was so intense he reportedly "blacked out" for a moment or two.

The history above is nearly all most astute chiropractors need to make a tentative diagnosis. What is yours? Also, what is the *arrow* directed towards in Fig. 3.8*A*, and is it of significance? Would you have altered the original treatment regime if you had been consulted initially?

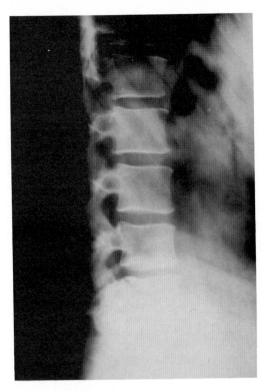

Fig. 3.8*B*. Andy B.

With the sudden onset, history and pattern of symptom expression you were correct if you tentatively identified an *acute lumbar disc syndrome*. What remains now is to confirm and locate.

A positive Lasegue's sign, Braggard's sign, stiff leg raising and dorsiflexion of the foot were achieved on the left. Marked paraspinal spasm was noted of the lower back and lumbosacral region.

Radiographs *A* and *B* of Fig. 3.8 indicate antalgic posture. Right lateral leaning with marked flattening of the lumbar lordosis is seen. Right lateral flexion of L4 on L5 is noted.

With antalgic posture, left sciatic neuropathy and right flexion subluxation of the segment above the lesion, it is possible to extrapolate that a prolapse or protrusion has occurred of the intervertebral disc at the L4-L5 level, with the lesion being located lateral to the nerve root on the left. It is well to remember that as a rule, if the lesion is located lateral to the nerve root, the patient will lean away from it (antalgic response), if it is medial to the nerve root, he will lean into the side of the neuropathy, and if it is a rare central lesion, he will bend forward at midline. The intent of antalgic response is to relieve the pressure and decompress the nerve root as much as possible (9, 25, 28). To enable plain film radiographic diagnosis of this condition, you must have antalgic posture, peripheral neuropathy and flexion malposition of the segment above. If any of the triad is missing, the diagnosis should be confirmed via CT scanning. (Myelographic examination is nearly extinct for this purpose in the up-to-date facility, thank heavens!)

The *arrow* in Fig. 3.8*A* is directed towards a pseudoforamen formed by the transverse process of L5, the sacral ala and the lateral margins of the facets. It is rarely of consequence, but we have heard reports of a nerve root becoming entrapped within. In this case it is an incidental finding.

Case 3.8

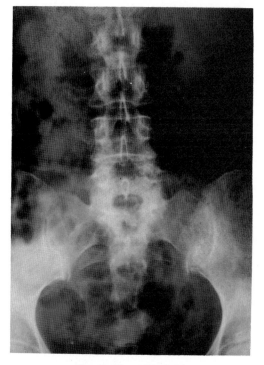

Fig. 3.9A.   Gloria V.

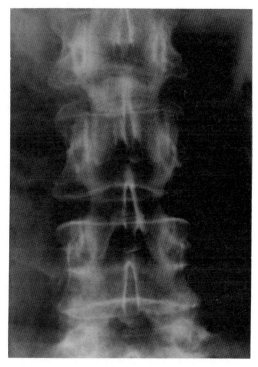

Fig. 3.9B.   Gloria V.

Gloria is a 63-year-old woman who has had a long history of repetitive lower back pain. Generally the complaint has revolved about the lumbosacral junction, from a combination of hyperextension activity and the effects of a rather pendulous abdomen.

These films (Fig. 3.9, *A* and *B*) were taken following a minor mishap, to exclude fracture. This was done. Our pattern of system review, however, noted a peculiar variation. It isn't seen often, and we would like to share it with you.

Once you have located the problem, answer these questions: Is this congenital, physiological or pathological? Will its presence have any long-lasting effects? Will treatment significantly alter its radiographic appearance, in time?

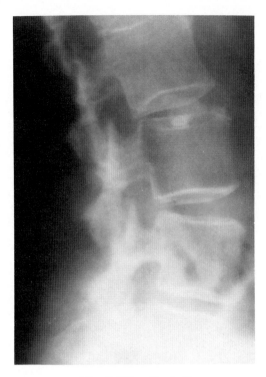

Fig. 3.9C.   Gloria V.

Total understanding of the *calcified nucleus pulposus* is lacking. While it is considered a dystrophic form of calcification, when seen in the adult it is usually of no clinical significance. In children, however, it is usually symptomatic. Of the various etiologies, only the idiopathic, posttraumatic and ochronosis forms involve the nucleus pulposus. All others affect the anulus fibrosus (12).

A significant characteristic of dystrophic calcification is the local alkalinity needed to precipitate the salts of calcium and phosphorus. This state of alkalinity is typically the result of devitalized tissue which has a lowered metabolic rate and carbon dioxide concentration. The causes may be physical or chemical, but each causes change in collagen that increases the affinity for calcium salts (12, 23).

From the above data we would antici-

pate frequent calcification of both the nucleus pulposus and anulus fibrosus, particularly in discal degeneration. This is not the case. Suggestion is made that perhaps sequestered or fragmented discal material is likely to be affected.

Note in Fig. 3.9C that a dense, ovoid radiopacity is seen at the L2-L3 disc space within the nucleus pulposus. Surrounding this density is a larger, less dense area whose total size can be judged by summation of both the AP and lateral views.

While questions remain about this form of physiological dystrophic calcification, we may assume that when found, it indicates a form of functional loss to the involved disc. Why loss of disc height is not characteristic is unknown. It is doubtful if any form of treatment can reverse this finding.

Case 3.9

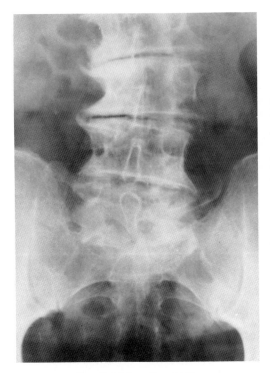

Fig. 3.10A. Gerald K.

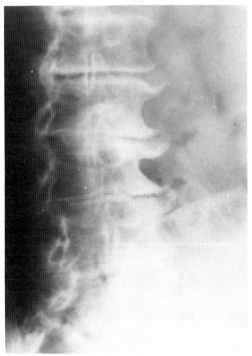

Fig. 3.10B. Gerald K.

Gerald is a 68-year-old man who has a history of chronic low back pain. The discovery radiographically (Fig. 3.10) of moderately severe lumbar discogenic spondylosis with a tendency towards ankylosis was not surprising. The dextrorotoscoliosis with concavity on the left and slight trapezoidal wedging of the L3 segment from right to left might have originally been compensatory to the large spatulated transverse process of L5 on the left.

The thin radiolucent streaking within the intervertebral disc spaces between L2-L3 and L3-L4 is referred to as the "*vacuum phenomenon.*" An old term, "phantom disc," was used to describe this entity when affecting the intervertebral disc, but as the same mechanism causes the effect in both joints and discs, the term is not often used at present (22). The exact pathophysiological mechanism responsible for the production of this radiolucent shadow is not fully understood. Some authorities believe that it represents a collection of lipid material within the degenerative disc, while others believe that the space becomes filled with gas derived from the blood or tissue fluids. When found in a degenerative disc, it is a constant finding. Most importantly, when the vacuum phenomenon is found, it is unequivocal evidence of degenerative disc disease regardless of other evidence, such as discal thinning, marginal thickening, sclerosis or spondylosis (9, 11, 20, 22).

Case 3.10

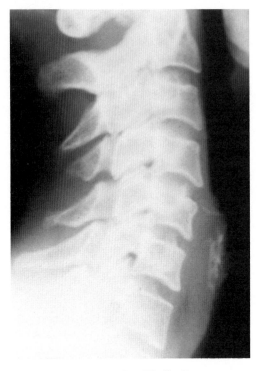

Fig. 3.11A. Phyllis C.

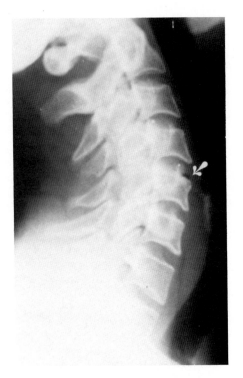

Fig. 3.11B. Phyllis C.

Phyllis is a 36-year-old woman who took a nasty spill while skiing about three weeks ago. Emergency room films taken at the time were negative for fracture, dislocation or osseous pathology. She was given a cervical collar to wear, along with muscle relaxants and pain medication. Diagnosis was "muscle spasm." After returning home from her vacation she continued to have pain and discomfort, particularly of the middle and lower cervical complex. The above films (Fig. 3.11, A and B) were taken. We included both flexion and extension views in this case due to the decrease of motor function and limited range of motion.

You will note that in the neutral view no significant abnormalities are noted. (C1 was cut off on the reproduction, not on the radiograph.) The extension view, however, demonstrates with a radiolucent "bubble" at the anterior portion of the C4-C5 intervertebral disc space. This represents a *vacuum phenomenon* but is etiologically unusual. While most radiolucent streaking seen in thinning intervertebral discs is the result of discal degeneration, this case represents posttraumatic gaseous or lipid entrapment, the result of cartilaginous damage, presumably from tearing or renting (9). It is likely that early or accelerated discal degeneration will occur at this level (27). The trauma sufficient to produce this degree of insult must have been significant. Even retrospectively it is difficult to see this finding on the neutral view alone.

SPONDYLOLISTHESIS

The forward movement of one vertebra on the one below is referred to as *spondylolisthesis*. With loss of continuity between the anterior and posterior sectors of the vertebral motor unit, the anchoring mechanism is lost, and forward displacement of the anterior sector may occur. It generally occurs at L5 but is not infrequently found in the upper segments of the lumbar spine.

The loss of anchoring is the result of spondylolysis or a defect in the pars interarticularis. This defect or fault represents a separation in the neural arch caused by a stress or fatigue fracture. While traumatic fractures do occur, the typical case of spondylolisthesis does not frequently present with a history of same. The separation of the pars is brought about by a continued cyclic backward bending movement. When spinal load is added, the weight is distributed through the intervertebral disc and posterior apophyseal joints. With repeated loading the disc tends to "creep" forward, increasing the backward bending movement of the segment, producing stress to the neural arch and pars. In time, a stress or fatigue fracture occurs. Additionally, spondylolytic fatigue fracture can occur in the fully flexed or partially flexed postures, provided that a cyclic loading situation is presented; walking for long periods of time with a heavy pack or bending forward continually lifting weights are examples (16).

With *bilateral pars defects* and forward displacement of the anterior portion of one vertebral segment, a spondylolytic spondylolisthesis occurs. While this forward displacement produces increased shearing to the disc with accelerated degeneration, herniation is rare. This presumably is due to the thickened and taut posterior longitudinal ligament which reinforces the anulus over the site of most herniations. Acute recurrent symptoms are frequent. A person with spondylolisthesis is 20 to 25 percent more likely to have significant back trouble during his life than one who does not (24). Frequently symptoms are due to postural stresses which produce the pincher effect (Fig. 3.13) to the attending soft tissues above and below the spondylolysis.

In *unilateral spondylolysis*, forward slipping or spondylolisthesis does not occur due to the intact opposite side maintaining its anchoring effect. Shearing of the disc is frequently severe, causing rapid degenerative breakdown and interarticular facet irritation on the normal side. When coupled with the pincher effect, this may produce more severe symptoms than when bilateral defects are present.

Nonspondylolytic spondylolisthesis may occur (Fig. 3.14B) in those instances of erosion changes to the zygapophyseal joints, i.e., posterior vertebral joint arthrosis and in association with elongation of the neural arch. The radiograph shows forward displacement, but no evidence of spondylolysis is seen. This form rarely exceeds a grade 1 classification (31).

Meyerding's classification of spondylolisthesis (Fig. 3.12F) is universally accepted. The sacral base is divided into quarters on the lateral film, and each is identified from posterior to anterior as 1, 2, 3 and 4. The alignment of the posterior-inferior corner of the forward-displaced segment above to the quarter sector below determines its "grade" (Fig. 3.12, A to E). In extreme displacement where total dislocation has occurred, a grade 5, 6 or higher may be arbitrarily designated.

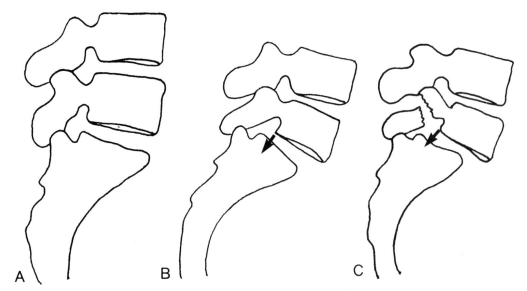

Fig. 3.12. *A:* Normal. *B:* Grade 1. *C:* Grade 2.

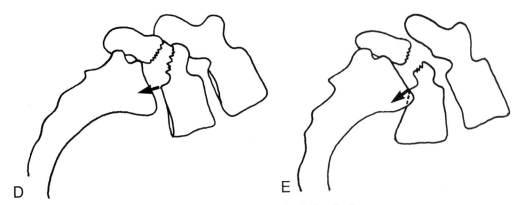

Fig. 3.12. *D:* Grade 3. *E:* Grade 4.

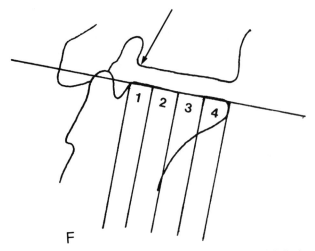

Fig. 3.12. *F:* Meyerding's classification of spondylolisthesis.

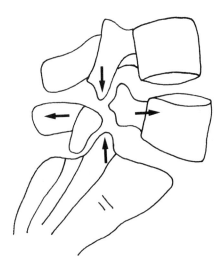

Fig. 3.13. Pincher effect.

In spondylolysis or a defect in the pars interarticularis, with or without spondylolisthesis, clinical symptoms are frequent. As the osseous fault frequently exists in the asymptomatic state as well, explanation as to the exacerbation of pain followed by spontaneous remission is required.

As can be seen in the drawing (Fig. 3.13), the gap or fault which remains following spondylolysis is subject to mechanical stress from the articular facets above and below. This intrusion into the gap causes irritation to the soft-tissue structures contained within. Swelling and edema may occur locally with resultant pain response. This response may produce reflex accommodation of the motor units above and below, often creating disrelationships of their articular facets—a "catch 22." The pain is typically localized and rarely produces nerve root involvement. When the swelling is reduced and positional disrelationships are corrected, if needed, symp-toms cease. The spondylolysis or gap remains. The patient must be advised to avoid excessive or heavy lifting and hyperextension of the lumbosacral complex—the most frequent cause of exacerbation. It may become necessary to utilize a lumbosacral support to restrict these activities. One of the more innocent yet damaging activities in this condition is overhead work, i.e., painting ceilings or eaves troughs, replacing light fixtures or bulbs, etc.

The fault is permanent. Exacerbation of symptom expression is frequent, unless precautions are exercised. During a state of remission, manipulation is directed towards increasing ligamentous integrity of the restraining groups and interarticular beds. Programmed exercises, including knee to chest, are often helpful in producing increased muscular tone and affording increased stability of the lumbosacral complex overall.

Case 3.11

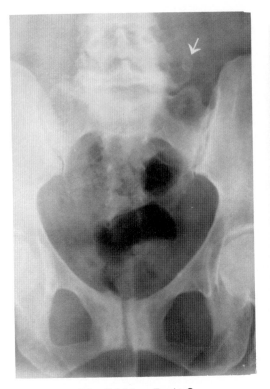

Fig. 3.14A. Rosie C.

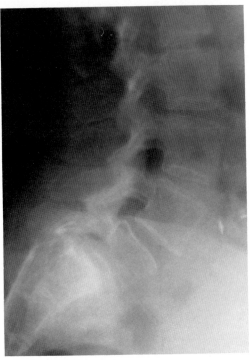

Fig. 3.14B. Rosie C.

Rosie, a 56-year-old black woman, had been overweight for most of her life. Her presenting complaints included frequent throbbing headache and constant low back pain, with periods of "heaviness" of both lower extremities. While the back pain was insidious, it was gradually worsening to a point where normal activity was being interfered with. She reported that even though she had had six children, her back ache now was worse than ever before.

The *arrow* in Fig. 3.14A represents a calcified retroperitoneal lymph node and does not enter into our discussion here.

Several conditions are of radiographic and clinical importance. One of these is quite common, albeit in this case not what you'd expect. The oblique films (on page 77) will help.

Rosie's headaches were due to hypertension, the result of her overweight and attending early glomerulonephritis.

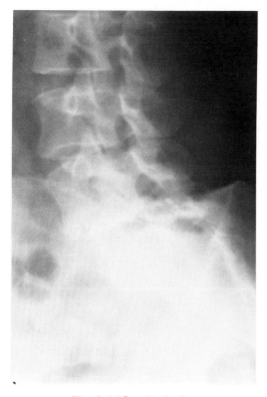

Fig. 3.14C. Rosie C.

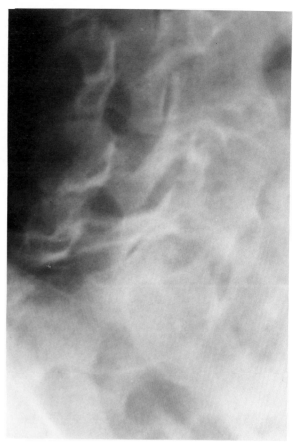

Fig. 3.14D. Rosie C.

In Fig. 3.14A, you will note a "soft" sclerotic thickening, typical of condensation, on either side of the pubic articulation. The interarticular joint space is narrowed, and no evidence of expansion or signs of contiguous architectural destruction is noted. This pattern is consistent with *osteitis condensans pubes*. In Rosie's case, it is related to multiple pregnancies and her pendulous abdomen.

In Fig. 3.14B, a dramatic anterior shift of Fergusson's weight-bearing line is noted with an apparent grade 2 spondylolisthesis of L5 on S1. As you will recall, in order to produce a grade 2 or more, a bilateral defect in the pars interarticularis or a spondylolysis must be present in a true spondylolisthesis. Examination of Fig. 3.14, C and D, indicates no such spondylolysis. Marked thinning, elongation and irregularity are seen of the pars bilaterally, but the "Scotty dog of LaChapele" is not wearing the characteristic collar indicating a pars defect. The forward displacement of L5 on S1 is the result of the architectural variations of the posterior articulating structures and not the result of spondylolysis. This formerly was referred to as "pseudospondylolisthesis" but currently and more descriptively is termed *nonspondylolytic spondylolisthesis*.

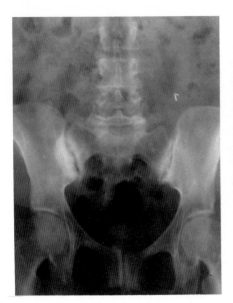

Fig. 3.14E. Rosie C.

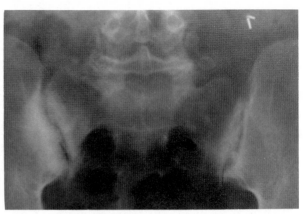

Fig. 3.14F. Rosie C.

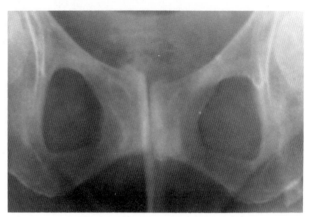

Fig. 3.14G. Rosie C.

It is now ten years later. Rosie continues to have recurrent low back and pelvic pain. Recent films (Fig. 3.14, E, F, and G) demonstrate significant radiographic evidence of chronicity. E and F present marked thickening and sclerosis of the left sacroiliac articulation. The vivid, increased radiolucent streaking is characteristic of the vacuum phenomenon of cartilaginous degeneration. When coupled with maintenance of interarticular joint space and sharpness of margination, acute inflammatory response can be ruled out. Thus, a chronic degenerative joint disease or, in this case, *chronic sacroiliac arthrosis* may be concluded. In Fig. 3.14G, the degree of osteitis condensans pubes, as was noted in

Fig. 3.14A, is diminished. Now seen is marginal thickening and sclerosis characteristic of joint arthrosis. Of interest is the alignment of the pubic articulation. Note the disruption of the pelvic ring due to superior displacement of the pubic ramus on the left. With this, concurrent posterior displacement of the left ilium would be anticipated. Attending stress to the left sacroiliac articulation is encountered with the resultant chronic degenerative joint disease or sacroiliac arthrosis as described. In case you are concerned, the degree of nonspondylolytic spondylolisthesis has not changed appreciably from that seen in Fig. 3.14B.

Case 3.12

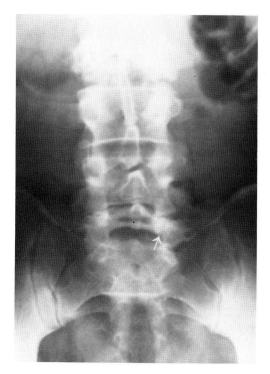

Fig. 3.15A. Robert J.

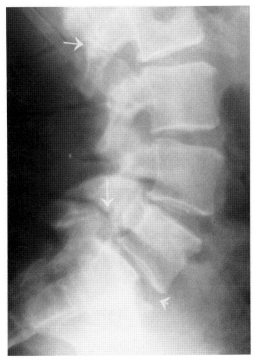

Fig. 3.15B. Robert J.

Robert is a roofer who fell from a ladder several weeks ago, landing on his buttock. Pain and deep aching are reported at the lumbosacral complex. Point tenderness is demonstrated at the L-S junction at midline. No neurological deficit is encountered, but a positive Lasegue's sign, Braggard's sign and stiff leg raising are seen. Residual discoloration of the right buttock is noted, the result of rather extensive contusion.

Historically, Robert has had frequent attacks of low back pain after carrying bundles of shingles. Two or three days of rest

have relieved the pain sufficiently to enable him to return to work. Many years ago he had seen his family physician who, after having films (x-rays) taken, told the patient he had a developmental anomaly but that it would never bother him. No treatment was given except for muscle relaxants.

The *arrows* in Fig. 3.15, *A* and *B*, which are directed towards the posterior motor units indicate what type of alteration? That directed to the sacral base draws your attention to a probable injury of what kind?

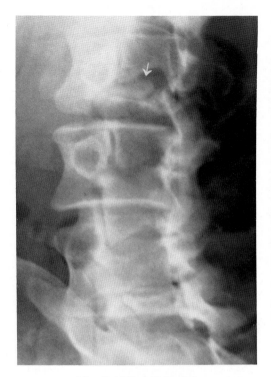

Fig. 3.15C. Robert J.

Fig. 3.15D. Robert J.

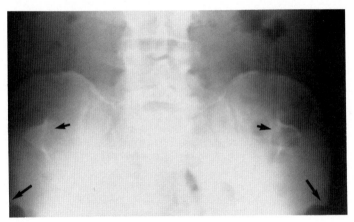

Fig. 3.15E. Robert J.

A grade 1 spondylolytic *spondylolisthesis* of L5 on S1 is seen. *Spondylolysis* of the pars interarticularis is noted of L5 and L2, bilaterally. The anterosuperior margin of the sacrum presents with a plate *fracture* with corner notching. Minimal bony debris is noted. The *arrows* in Fig. 3.15, C and D, show small *intercalary* or *ectopic bone* formation. All findings except the sacral fracture present with no evidence to suggest recent development. The various biomechanical disrelationships with al-

tered weight bearing are obvious.

An incidental finding on Robert's film is bilateral *iliac horns* (Fig. 3.15E). Typically this finding is of little clinical concern. However, when associated with a beaking contour pointed inferiorly of the iliac crests, it may indicate the presence of the HOOD (hereditary onychoosteodysplasia) syndrome. The iliac horns are osteocartilaginous exostoses. They may also occur as an isolated finding in Fong's disease (12).

Case 3.13

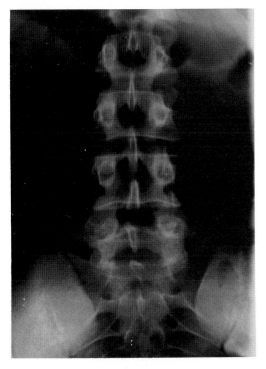

Fig. 3.16A. Gordon G.

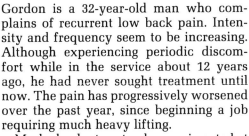

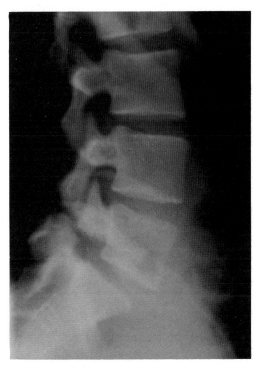

Fig. 3.16B. Gordon G.

Gordon is a 32-year-old man who complains of recurrent low back pain. Intensity and frequency seem to be increasing. Although experiencing periodic discomfort while in the service about 12 years ago, he had never sought treatment until now. The pain has progressively worsened over the past year, since beginning a job requiring much heavy lifting.

Marked palpatory tenderness is noted at the lumbosacral and L4-L5 interspace at midline. No radiation, paresthesias, mus-cular atrophy or positive neurological findings were recorded.

The AP radiograph (Fig. 3.16A) suggests a facet tropism at L4-L5, i.e., coronal on the left and sagittal on the right. This, however, appears only contributory to the more serious condition demonstrated on the lateral film (Fig. 3.16B). Can you identify and classify this condition? Are other films necessary for confirmation? Which ones?

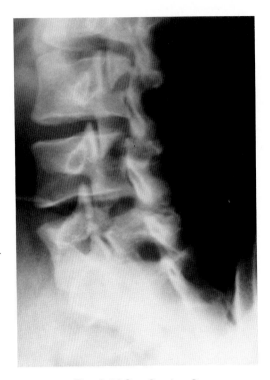

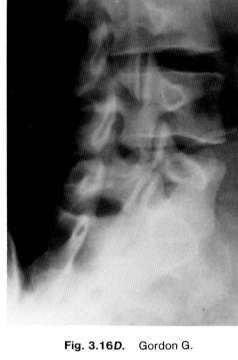

Fig. 3.16C. Gordon G.   **Fig. 3.16D.** Gordon G.

While the area of spondylolysis or defect in the pars interarticularis of L5 is well demonstrated on the lateral view (Fig. 3.16B), the oblique views (Fig. 3.16, C and D) are often taken to verify and confirm this diagnosis. As noted in these films, the "Scotty dog's neck" is broken, or it is wearing a collar. The latter two descriptive terms are used to describe the pars defect or spondylolysis. This finding coupled with the anterolisthesis or forward displacement of the L5 anterior segment on the sacrum is conclusive evidence of a *grade 1 spondylolytic spondylolisthesis.*

Discussion of the etiology, clinical expression and importance of this condition is found elsewhere in this text. In this case, as in so many similar to it, symptom expression is dependent upon soft-tissue insult, the result of the "pincher effect" caused by occupational stress and postural fatigue. Treatment is conservative, i.e., manipulation coupled with direct and clear instruction in appropriate lifting, bending, twisting and other postural attitudes. Occasionally, employment of a lumbosacral support is of great value.

Case 3.14

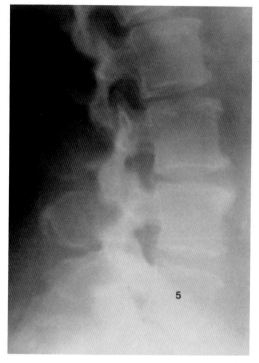

Fig. 3.17A. John K.

John is 49 years old, although his spine looks much older (Fig. 3.17A).

He complains of chronic low back ache with stiffness. As his job requires a great deal of overhead reaching and stretching as well as bending and lifting, he seems always to have a backache.

No sharp pain, paresthesias, muscular atrophy or positive neurological findings were recorded.

After reviewing the films with the patient, it was learned that for nearly 20 years he had ridden a motorcycle and had participated in many hill climbs. He suffered several broken bones (leg, foot and arm) after being "thrown" from his machine.

Two conditions are demonstrated in John's low back. One is a frequently seen and clinically significant condition. The other is less well known but is of importance in explaining the cause and effect of his present complaint.

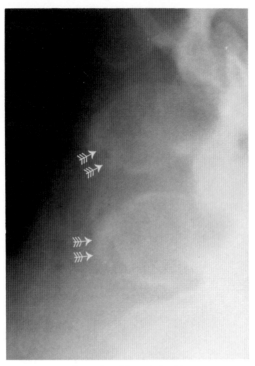

Fig. 3.17B.   John K.

The *lumbar spondylosis* involving L2, L3 and L4 is evident via multiple osteophytic spur formations. Slight distal thinning is noted between L3 and L4 (Fig. 3.17A).

Additionally, you will note the *calcific infiltrate* at the attachment site of the intraspinous and supraspinous ligaments into the spinous processes of L3 and L4 (see *arrows* on Fig. 3.17B). This finding indicates prior insertional stress and/or injury with resultant loss of integrity and resiliency.

The combination of these findings, i.e., both anterior and posterior involvement of the motor unit(s), indicates probable hypomobility and fixation between L3 and L4. Limitation of excursion and/or moto-ricity produces abnormal stress to the articular facets during the extremes of both flexion and extension movement, causing capsular stress and/or irritation. This explains John's chronic repetitive complaint.

Had you considered the changes of the spinous process attachments as Baastrup's disease, you would have had plenty of company. Baastrup's disease or "kissing spinous processes," however, is a condition of marginal arthrosis of the spinous processes, should they happen to abut or make chronic repetitive contact with each other. The marginal thickening and sclerosis involves the spinous processes themselves, and calcific infiltrate into the ligamentous attachments is not characteristic.

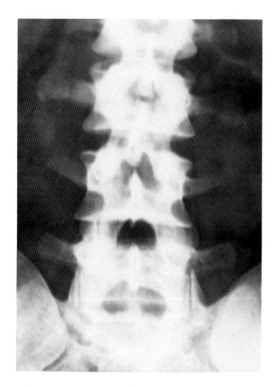

Fig. 3.18A. Sagittal facet facings at L5-S1.

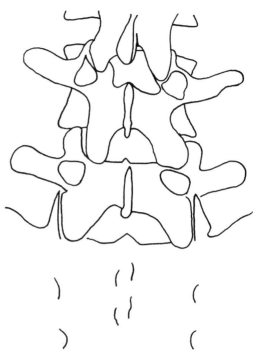

Fig. 3.18B. Schematic of Fig. 3.18A demonstrates, at L5-S1, sagittal facet facings considered the most stable.

With the lower lumbar spine, it is critically important to know that the overall prognosis in a given case may well center about the spine's anatomical stability. Understanding the interarticular facet structures is a must. Except for discal lesions and nerve root entrapment, few other conditions present as frequently for treatment as facet synovitis of the lumbosacral complex.

No other level of the spine receives, or is designed to receive, the work load in man that the lumbosacral junction receives. This motor unit distributes its load near equally between the intervertebral disc and the posterior articular facets. Ap-

proximately 40 to 50 percent of the torque strength of the joint is supplied by the posterior structures, i.e., 40 percent by the facets, 10 percent by the ligaments. The remaining 50 percent is born by the disc and annular fibers. The anatomical orientation of the interarticular facets must be bilaterally symmetrical to prevent rapid breakdown of the annular fibers and to provide necessary protection for the intervertebral disc (24). The majority of people present with sagittal facet facings from L1 through L4 and coronal facings at L5-S1. Variations in activity and stress therefore govern the clinical significance of the facet facings.

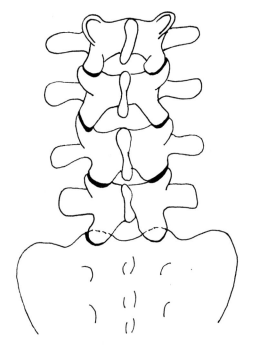

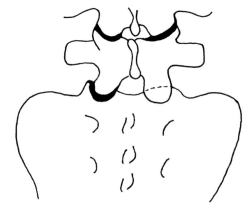

Fig. 3.18G. Facet tropism. Sagittal on the left, coronal on the right (L5-S1).

Fig. 3.18C. Bilateral coronal facet facings considered the most unstable.

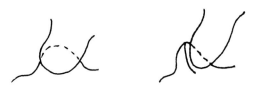

Fig. 3.18D. Coronal. **Fig. 3.18E.** Sagittal.

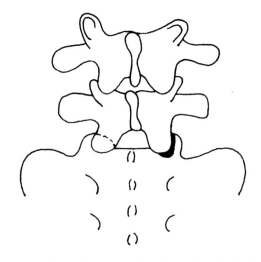

Fig. 3.18H. Facet tropism. Coronal on the left, sagittal on the right (L5-S1).

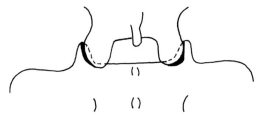

Fig. 3.18F. Bilateral semisagittal facets. Stable.

When both facets are oriented in a *sagittal* direction (Fig. 3.18, *A* and *B*), there is less torque, and flexion-extension motions are uninhibited. This is considered the *most* stable of the facet facings at L5-S1 (20, 24). In the event that both facets are symmetrical, although in a coronal direction, rotation is not inhibited, but the cam action of flexion-extension is nearly absent (Fig. 3.18C and 3.19). In man this is referred to as the most unstable of the L5-

S1 facet facings and may help to explain the relatively high incidence of lower back pain associated with modern day activities.

Facet tropism, referring to a tendency to turn towards or away from, refers to the facing of the facet in relation to its counter part on the opposite side. Typically of most significance at the L5-S1 level, the facets will present with coronal facing on one side and sagittal facing on the other (Fig. 3.18, *G* and *H*). Note: Tropism has been referred to as facet asymmetry. We agree that it does represent a form of asymmetry. For ease in understanding, however, it is practical to use the term tropism exclusively when referring to the facet facings and their orientation to each other, saving the term asymmetry for use in describing variation in size and shape of the facets or articular processes.

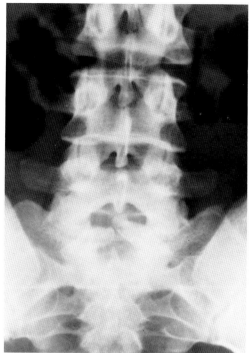

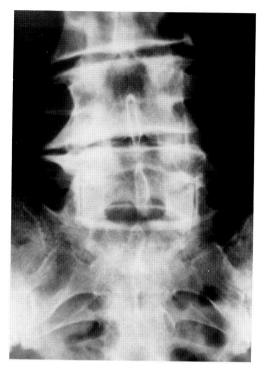

Fig. 3.19. Bilateral coronal facet facings at L5-S1. Unstable. (Note spina bifida occulta at S1.)

Fig. 3.20. Facet tropism L4-L5.

Before leaving the discussion of facet tropism, a few salient points are needed. The more obliquely orientated the facet, the less mechanically suited it is to resist rotation. When one facet is rotated against its fellow, the joint is forced apart on that side—a frequent cause of acute synovial insult. Repetition may produce early degenerative changes within the facets, i.e., arthrosis. The effects of the facet rotation towards the side of the oblique facet combine to produce maximal strain on the posterior lateral angle of the anulus fibrosus, a frequent site of discal rupture. A high correlation has been demonstrated between the side of the disc prolapse and the side of the more obliquely oriented facet (24, 25) (Fig. 3.20).

The lumbar discs will tolerate flexion and extension much better than rotational stresses. The posterior facets protect the disc from rotational stresses. When surgical removal or agenesis of one facet occurs, rotational instability results with subsequent rapid degeneration of the disc.

Clinical management in tropism must include instruction to the patient as to which movements he must avoid in order to reduce mechanical stress. For instance, we know that coronal facet facings are not consistent with flexion-extension activity; ergo, in the case of bilateral coronal facets, this activity must be restricted. In tropism, guarded movements of this type, particularly on the side of coronal facings, are necessary. In general, facet tropism limits the degree and amount of hyperextension, hyperflexion and lateral bending of the lumbosacral complex.

Case 3.15

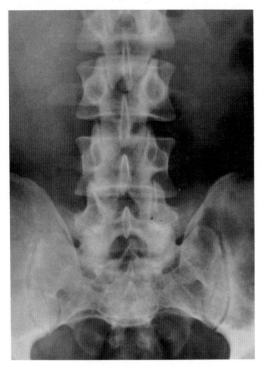

Fig. 3.21A. Tom S.

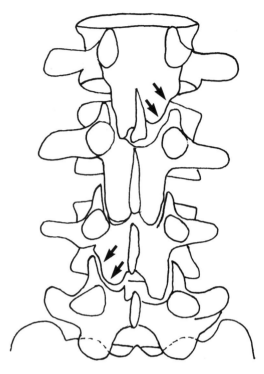

Fig. 3.21B. Schematic of Fig. 3.21A.

In the understanding of spinal biomechanics the significance of architectural symmetry is of prime importance. The bodily adaptation and compensation mechanisms, while truly amazing in their ability, are nonetheless governed by inherent limitations. As the upright posture of man requires that the interarticular facet structures provide for accommodation of movement and range as well as support, their size, shape and symmetry determine this ability.

While true symmetry is lacking of any two anatomical structures, i.e., the one hand being larger than the other, etc., the closest approximation of symmetry is ideally required of the spinal structures to avoid disturbance of biomechanical rhythm with resultant altered function.

In the case of Tom S. (Fig. 3.21) the inferior articular processes of L4 on the left and of L2 on the right are each asymmetrical in their size, shape and form. Each present with *facet asymmetry*. Fortunately in this case the overall disturbance of spinal motoricity and rhythm is minimized due to the counterbalance provided, i.e., one shortened on the left, the other on the right. If only one side had been involved, the proprioceptive righting reflex would have been activated, causing compensation to occur with altered spinal rhythm and balance the result.

It is important not only to recognize the facet asymmetry and to determine what effect this has on spinal biomechanics but also to differentiate this from facet tropism which has a greater localized effect on spinal rhythm and segmental function.

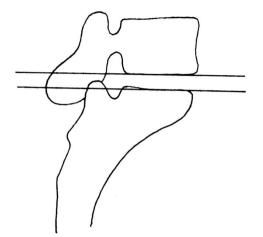

Fig. 3.22A. Normal.

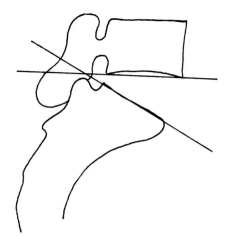

Fig. 3.22B. Facet syndrome.

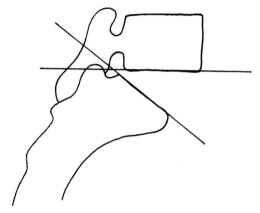

Fig. 3.22C. Facet syndrome.

The *facet syndrome* is a frequently encountered radiographic finding. Because it is considered the result of various etiological factors, it is rarely considered an entity in itself. Perhaps this explains the relative dearth of information in the literature.

In order to determine its presence, the lumbosacral angle is employed—a line drawn across the sacral base and another along the inferior body plate margin of L5. These two lines normally bisect well behind the intervertebral foramina (IVF) at approximately a 5- to 12-degree angle. Variations within normal limits do occur. The key word is BEHIND the IVF (15).

When the lines bisect at the posterior margin of the IVF (Fig. 3.22B) or within it (Fig. 3.22C), biomechanical disrelationships of importance are present.

Hyperextension subluxation of L5, retrolisthesis of L5, anteflexion of the sac-

rum, discal thinning with creep of its internal matrix, erosion of the posterior articular facets, and others may all produce this increase of the lumbosacral angle.

Of clinical significance is the interarticular facet imbrication or telescoping which occurs. This alteration causes synovial irritation, capsular strain and segmental adaptation, including alteration of the attending IVF. With time these changes may produce thickening, sclerosis and marginal irregularity of facet arthrosis. Its effect on degeneration of the disc and annular fibers due to the increased torsional stress will compound any existing problem.

In a clinically expressive facet syndrome, care should be taken not only to treat the current symptoms but also to determine its cause and institute those procedures necessary to deter recurrence.

Section 4

Common Arthritides

Case 4.1

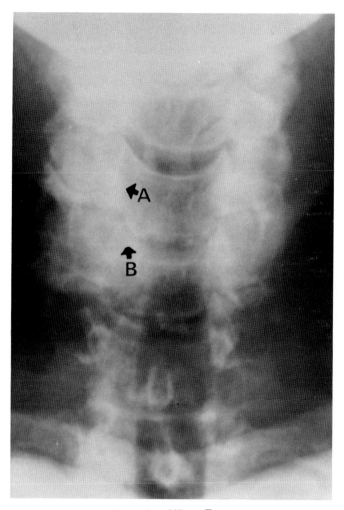

Fig. 4.1. Allison T.

Allison T. complains of chronic, recurrent stiffness and ache in the left side of the neck, accompanied by frequent headaches. The presence of paresthesias in the upper extremities is denied. After review of Fig. 4.1, would you suspect any significant vertigo?

Arrow A in Fig. 4.1 points to marked thickening, sclerosis and marginal irregularity of the zygapophyseal articulation. Note the proliferative extension laterally from the joint margin typical of osteophytosis. This condition is referred to as *posterior vertebral joint arthrosis* and is frequently accompanied by fixation with loss of interbody mobility. *Arrow B* directs the eye towards the covertebral joint of Luschka which shows *no* evidence of arthrosis. By its absence, it is suggested that the vertebral artery is not compromised and therefore there should be no significant vertigo from vascular insufficiency.

Case 4.2

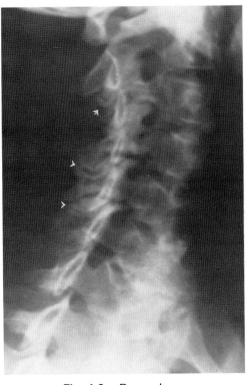

Fig. 4.2. Renae J.

Fig. 4.2 is another example of *posterior vertebral joint arthrosis (PVJA)*. Unlike the PVJA of Allison T. (Fig. 4.1), however, the PVJA of Renae J. (Fig. 4.2) is not as advanced. Early proliferative outgrowth, marginal irregularity and sclerosis are noted (*arrows*). Alterations of the intervertebral foramina are seen, particularly between C3 and C4, due to proliferative extension of the zygapophyseal articulations, coupled with attending positional disrelationships. Neurovascular entrapment or compromise is problematical.

Case 4.3

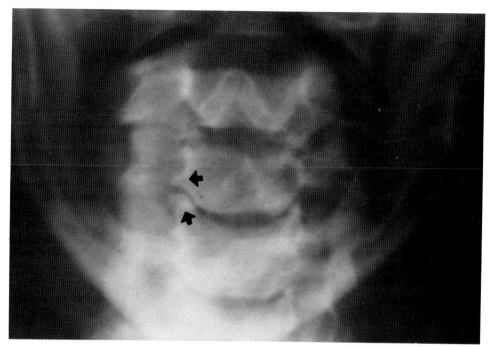

Fig. 4.3. Janice B.

Janice is a 47-year-old woman who complains of vertigo, headache and pain on lateral bending or hyperextension of the head on the neck. After review of Fig. 4.3, would you associate the symptom complex with neurological or vascular involvement, and would it be transient or constant?

The covertebral joints of Luschka found only in the cervical spine are of clinical significance when they have undergone the thickening, sclerosis and marginal irregularity of arthrosis. Due to the proximity of these joints to the vertebral artery which lies just lateral to them, the hypertrophic changes may encroach on the artery with resultant compromise of its diameter (8).

In Fig. 4.3 the *arrows* are directed towards two early osteophytic proliferative changes involving the covertebral joints between C3 and C4 on the left. The degree of change in this case is very early but clearly demonstrates the proliferative extension which typically extends laterally toward the vertebral artery channel.

Even in this case of *early covertebral joints of Luschka arthrosis* the integrity of the vertebral artery must always be considered. Should atherosclerosis render the vessel friable or less resilient than normal, vigorous manipulation via a "breaking" technique, i.e., with the head turned laterally and the neck hyperextended, may be contraindicated.

This patient's symptoms are transient in nature and related to pure biomechanical insult via encroachment of the vertebral artery and attending vascular insufficiency, with positioning of the head and neck.

Case 4.4

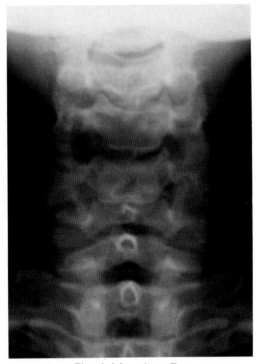

Fig. 4.4A. Jean E.

Jean is a 40-year-old woman who has developed moderate stiffness and ache of the lower neck with extension into her shoulders bilaterally. She reports that her hands "fall asleep" easily and tend to be cold. No loss of grip strength, swelling or finger joint pain is noted. Lately she awakens with a basilar headache which dissipates spontaneously after an hour of activity.

Her history is essentially unremarkable, although she does report striking her head following a fall from a horse when she was about 20.

Orthopedic, neurological and laboratory findings are of questionable value.

Because this clinical presentation is so typical of patients seeking the help of their chiropractor, it is included. It is certainly not a "toughie," and your clinical expertise should not be overly taxed. Several questions might make it interesting. From review of Fig. 4.4A, what classification of subluxation might be expected? Are the covertebral joints of Luschka involved? Is vertebral artery compromise suspect? In addition to manipulation, what other ancillary procedures would you employ? What is your prognostication and recommendations to the patient? What significant clinical findings will alert you and the patient to deterioration of the condition, should it occur?

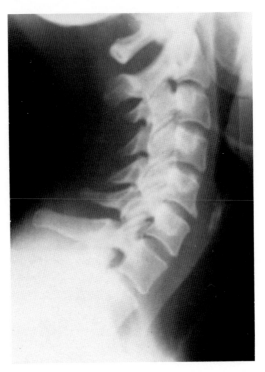

Fig. 4.4B.   Jean E.

The decreased interosseous spacing subluxation at C5–C6 is apparent in Fig. 4.4B. A small osteophytic spur formation is noted at the anterior-inferior contiguous body plate margin of C5. The posterior-inferior margin is also suspect. These findings are consistent with *early cervical discogenic spondylosis.*

The covertebral joints of Luschka demonstrate with decrease of interarticular joint spacing but with no evidence of marginal arthrosis. No vertebral artery compromise would be suspect.

The present symptoms are related to the loss of motoricity, i.e., hypomobility, fixation and altered cervical rhythm, the result of discal degeneration. During the resting state, contraction of the capsular ligaments and muscles occurs, presumably a protective reflex.

Due to the inability of the degenerative disc to undergo complete restoration by imbibition, the hysteresis or shock absorbability of the viscoelastic disc is decreased (26). Stiffness is encountered upon awakening. Relaxation of the capsular structure occurs after minimal exercise, producing relief.

With manipulation, it is hoped that a decrease in the rate of discal degeneration will occur due to increased vascularity, imbibition and ligamentous integrity. The degenerative process will proceed, however, and in time the degree and amount of decreased interosseous spacing and spondylosis will produce foraminal alteration, with or without spur intrusion. Neurovascular entrapment is of greatest concern. The patient should be instructed to report any paresthesias or numbness immediately so that reevaluation may be undertaken.

Ancillary measures utilized during the various stages of conservative manipulative management include physiotherapy, the use of a cervical pillow, and overhead cervical traction.

Case 4.5

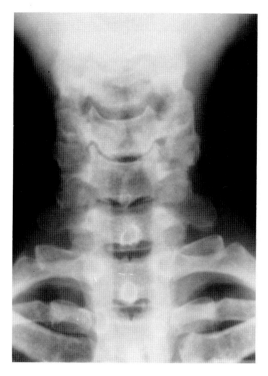

Fig. 4.5A.   Alice M.

Sometimes we get caught up in the more dramatic and overlook the obvious.

Alice, a 32-year-old housewife, has recently noticed stiffness and ache of the lower neck and shoulder when arising in the morning. She has stopped using a pillow when sleeping, and the complaint, although still present, is not as severe.

Clinical examination indicates moderate hypomobility of the lower cervical complex with motion palpation. Hyperextension of the head on the neck is slightly restricted due to discomfort. No other positive findings are noted with neurological, orthopedic or laboratory testing.

Historically, Alice relates a minor rear end collision approximately six years ago, for which no treatment was undertaken. She remembers some stiffness and ache of the neck which dissipated within a week. She has had no complaint since, until the past three or four months.

Your review of Fig. 4.5A should direct you not only to the level of the problem but, with the history above, give you a running start on your tentative diagnosis.

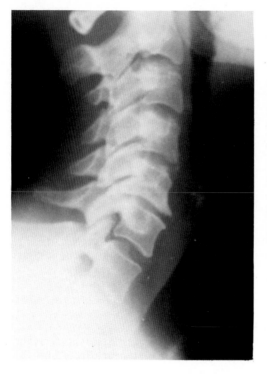 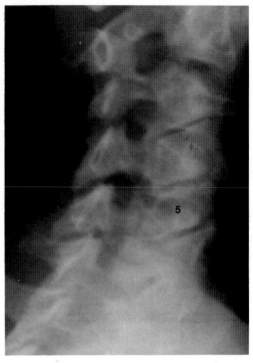

Fig. 4.5B. Alice M.   **Fig. 4.5C.** Alice M.

The decrease of interosseous spacing involving both the intervertebral disc space and the covertebral joints of Luschka is apparent between C5 and C6 in Fig. 4.5A. In Fig. 4.5B, this same thinning of the intervertebral disc is the result of *early moderate discal degeneration*. Note the small, early osteophytic spur formation from the anterolateral contiguous body plate margins. While no definitive foraminal encroachment due to spur intrusion is noted in Fig. 4.5C, foraminal alteration due to the positional disrelationship between C5 and C6 is seen. Neurovascular entrapment or compromise is doubtful.

While discal thinning may be due to hypoplasia or underdevelopment in growth, this rarely produces contiguous sclerosis, thickening or marginal irregularity commensurate with discal degeneration and spondylosis.

Alice does well with periodic manipulation of the cervical spine. An orthopedic pillow, i.e., a contoured pillow, is employed for sleeping comfort while stabilizing the cervical lordosis. Should time cause an increase in the degree and amount of discogenic spondylosis, utilization of overhead traction might prove beneficial. The advent of paresthesias of either upper extremity could herald osteophytic spur intrusion into the intervertebral foramina.

Case 4.6

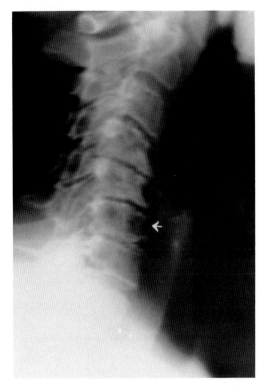

Fig. 4.6A. Ross J.

Ross J. has had marked stiffness and limited range of motion of the head and neck for years, following a severe automobile accident.

While no cervical fractures were uncovered at the time, rather extensive soft-tissue injury to both the muscles and ligaments was present. Treatment at the time included immobilization and physiotherapy.

No infectious or neoplastic involvement was noted in his history.

Since the accident, an insidious recurrent paresthesia has developed in the right forearm and hand. His limited range of motion is painless except for occasional basilar headache.

Can you identify the condition(s) now present, describe the cervical lordosis, indicate the levels of mobility and/or hypomobility, pinpoint the probable cause of paresthesia, and prognosticate the probable sequelae? Also, what significance do you attach to the radiolucent area located in the anterior one third of the C6 vertebral body (*arrow* on Fig. 4.6A)? Don't forget to look at all the laterals before answering!

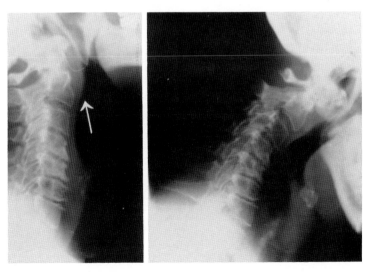

Fig. 4.6B. Ross J.

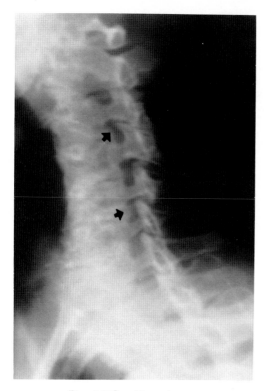

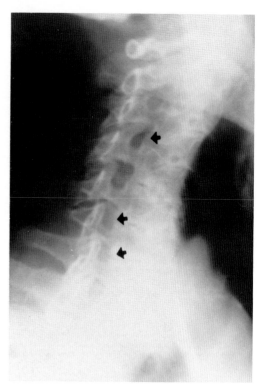

Fig. 4.6C. Ross J.

Fig. 4.6D. Ross J.

The lordosis is markedly reversed owing to marked flattening below C4, hyperflexion malposition of C4, and forward displacement of the head and neck above. Discal thinning with attending marginal irregularity and osteophytic proliferative spur formation is noted of their contiguous body plate margins from C4 through C7. This finding is consistent with *discogenic spondylosis*. You will note that spur intrusion is now beginning (at the *arrows* of Fig. 4.6, *C* and *D*), particularly at C5–C6 and C6–C7 on the right. This finding has produced the insidious paresthesia due to neurovascular entrapment or compromise.

The flexion-extension views (Fig. 4.6*B*) indicate that marked hypomobility and fixation is present below C4. Nearly all motion or mobility occurs above C4. Due to this transitional level of fixed versus mobile intersegmented circumstance, a positional disrelationship, i.e., subluxation, is noted at C3–C4 with attending foraminal alterations (*upper arrows* of Fig. 4.6, *C* and *D*). Neurovascular entrapment here is doubtful.

The radiolucent area of the anterior C6 segment is due to architectural variation, presumably due to the previous trauma, which has produced a localized area of osteoporosis. You will note that no deformity in height of the segment or loss of the anterior vertebral margin is present. In fact, small osteophytes have taken origin from this margin. By the way, we did a double take too, 'cause it sure did look like osteolytic destruction, particularly on the neutral lateral.

Case 4.7

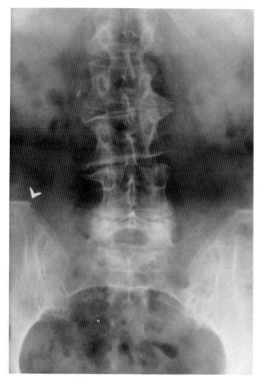

Fig. 4.7A. Robert M.

Robert has experienced chronic low back stiffness and bone ache which has never completely gone away. In fact it has progressively worsened over the past few years. Some lumbar flank and groin discomfort has also been noted.

Following an episode of lifting cut logs from his truck and carrying them to his wood pile, he developed an acute sharp pain in the left L-S region with no paresthesias into the lower extremities.

What is your impression of the cause for the chronic recurrent problem? Is ankylosis present? What subluxations are a part of this complex in this case? Will you attempt to markedly alter their disrelationships or attempt to inhibit further progression? Maintain and perhaps restore interjoint mobility? Is the alteration present at the *white arrowhead* in Fig. 4.7A of diagnostic significance?

Given Robert's history, do you see evidence in Fig. 4.7A of a probable acute lesion, or do you feel an exacerbation of the chronic alteration is responsible?

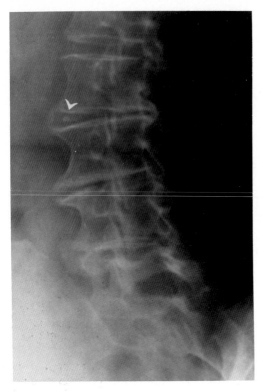

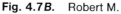

Fig. 4.7B. Robert M.

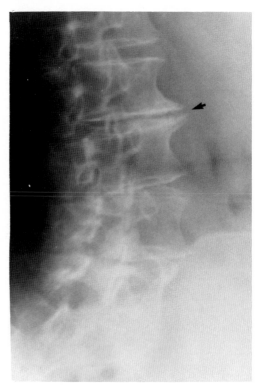

Fig. 4.7C. Robert M.

Discogenic ankylosing spondylosis is not an infrequent form of chronic low back pain. The ankylosis is typically the result of the healing phase of an inflammatory process. With it comes hypomobility of the involved segment(s). While specific etiology remains obscure, the localized segmental involvement suggests a posttraumatic or stress adaptation inflammatory response.

Careful review of Fig. 4.7, B and C, in Bob's case suggests that while a definite attempt towards ankylosis is ongoing, it is not yet complete. Thus, while mobility is already limited, complete fixation has not been attained. The *white arrowhead* in Fig. 4.7B indicates a small calcific infiltrate into the anterolateral portion of the intervertebral disc (IVD) on the left, the result of prior discal insult and/or injury. Manipu-

lation is aimed at maintaining and perhaps increasing interjoint mobility, thus inhibiting further progression of the ankylosing process. Once the ankylosis formation is complete, an attempt to break or loosen the fixation is contraindicated. The oblique radiographs of Fig. 4.7, B and C, also indicate interarticular facet imbrication (telescoping), particularly on the left (RAO, Fig. 4.7B). Interarticular facet synovitis and/or irritation is suspect and represents the site of Bob's acute symptoms. The *white arrowhead* seen in Fig. 4.7A shows thickening and sclerosis at the attachment site of the ileotransverse (iliolumbar) ligament and indicates prior local periosteitis, the result of insertional stress. This is often found in cases of the chronic unstable low back syndrome.

Case 4.8

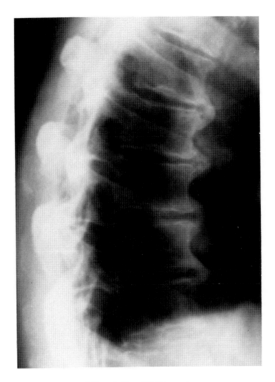

Fig. 4.8. William S.

Bill is a 57-year-old experimental laboratory chief who has developed sharp pain in the midthoracic region. While he has reportedly had ache and stiffness for years, these have not interfered with his daily routine until now.

A moderate thoracic kyphosis with inability to stand straight is noted. Bill relates that he feels fairly comfortable when standing but, after sitting for a few minutes, develops sharp pain in the midthoracic spine near midline on the right. Some pain radiates towards the periphery along the posterior T6 rib on the right. He reports that it feels as though someone is "sticking a knife" from his back to the front of his chest on the right, particularly when coughing or sneezing.

Marked muscular rigidity is found throughout the paravertebral structures of the thoracic spine bilaterally. Point tenderness is noted at T6–T8 on the right. The thorax is somewhat bell-shaped due to limited respiratory excursion associated with the kyphosis.

Pain began after a severe cold with much coughing and sneezing about four weeks ago. It seemed worsened after shoveling snow a few days ago. Neurological and orthopedic testing was essentially negative. No laboratory work was done.

The acute symptoms are related to an acute thoracocostal facet subluxation at T6 on the right. This rib lesion is not demonstrated on this film. The history is characteristic for the production of a thoracocostal facet lesion and is detected by careful physical examination. Fortunately this lesion responds quickly to manipulation (29, 30).

Fig. 4.8 provides evidence of underlying pathology which explains chronicity. This condition has produced the kyphosis and limitation in range of motion throughout the thoracic spine. What is it? Can manipulation be of help, and if so, should an attempt be made to alter those changes of the anterior motor units noted?

Case 4.9

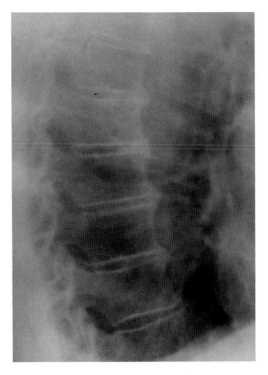

Fig. 4.9. George F.

George is a 61-year-old attorney. Like William (Fig. 4.8) he has marked stiffness throughout the thoracic spine. No sharp pain is usually experienced, but a limitation of flexibility occasionally interferes with some activity. He is anxious to get "loosened up," as he is planning a golf vacation.

In both cases the changes and alterations are predominately thoracic. Only minimal evidence of the condition is present in the cervical and lumbar regions. This localized involvement is typical, although certainly not restricted. It does help in differentiation from the lumbosacral involvement of ankylosing spondylitis.

You will note that both William (Fig. 4.8) and George (Fig. 4.9) have decrease in height of the intervertebral discs throughout. Marginal sclerosis and thickening of the vertebral end plates is noted more in William's case. Both present with osteophytic spurring from the anterolateral margins which are predominately horizon-

tal in direction. This distinguishes these from the vertical direction found in the syndesmophytic formation of rheumatoid arthritis. The osteophytic proliferative spur formations tend towards joining together, i.e., ankylosis. While it is doubtful that total fusion or ankylosis has occurred by the osteophytes themselves, cartilaginous attachment is probable, and therefore the condition is termed chronic thoracic discogenic spondylosis with tendency towards ankylosis. Some would prefer *ankylosing spondylosis.* The condition must always be differentiated from ankylosing spondylitis.

Manipulation is of benefit in these cases by producing a "freeing up" or loosening of the capsular fixation of the posterior motor unit. This allows for some increase of motoricity, lessened synovial irritation and increased blood flow. Vigorous manipulative procedures aimed at "breaking" the ankylosis is contraindicated.

Case 4.10

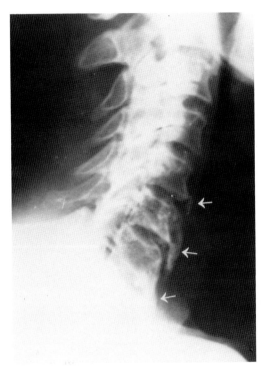

Fig. 4.10A. Gus Y.

Gus is a 73-year-old former plumber who has had stiffness in his neck for years. Occasional headache and a sharp "twinge" of pain with lateral bending and hyperextension of the neck are reported.

Recently he noticed some difficulty in deglutition, claiming some foods seem to "stick in his throat."

Orthopedic examination indicates limited range of motion, particularly in hyperflexion and lateral bending of the cervical spine. Marked muscular rigidity is noted paravertebrally, but no point tenderness is exhibited. Neurological examination was unrevealing.

It is important to differentiate between an osteophytic and syndesmophytic formation. Typically the osteophyte is associated with degenerative disc or joint disease and extends outward from the vertebra or joint margin. The syndesmophyte is typical of ankylosing spondylitis and tends to bridge the joint interspace in a vertical fashion. In both of these conditions the intervertebral or interarticular joint spacing is found to be thinned.

In Gus' case there appears to be a paradoxical situation. The large calcific structures (see *arrows* in Fig. 4.10A) are bridging the interspaces, but the disc space appears normal. In addition, Gus also suffers from a concurrent condition found in the aged. Now, let's test your memory. I'll give you a hint by telling you that when this condition invades spinal areas in addition to the cervical spine or when more than four continuous segments are involved, it is sometimes referred to as diffuse idiopathic skeletal hyperostosis or DISH.

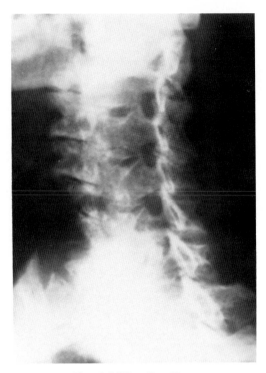

Fig. 4.10*B*.   Gus Y.

An exuberant osteophytosis is the term used to describe *Forestier's disease* or ankylosing hyperostosis. Generally found in the aged, it is often asymptomatic. Due to its predilection for the lower cervical and upper thoracic spine, it may cause increase of the thoracic kyphosis. When extensive or erratic, the osteophytes tend to encroach into the posterior esophagus and cause difficult swallowing, particularly when the bolus is large or firm.

Representing extensive ossification around degenerative cartilage, with involvement of both the anterior longitudinal ligament and annular fibers, the exuberant osteophytosis tends to bridge the intervertebral disc. This may at times be confused with the syndesmophytic for-mations of ankylosing spondylitis, but the absence of characteristic change in the lumbosacral spine and sacroiliac joints in this latter condition is of differential significance (7, 11, 18).

Of the more important characteristics are the absence of degenerative disc thinning and the clear identification of the vertebral corners, both of which are typical of osteophytosis found in discogenic spondylosis.

In Gus' case a concurrent posterior vertebral joint arthrosis is evidenced by marginal thickening, sclerosis and proliferative extension of the zygapophyseal articulations. This PVJA is not typical of Forestier's disease.

Case 4.11

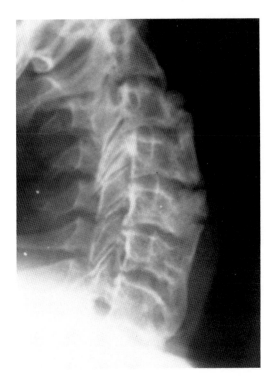

Fig. 4.11 A. John W.

John is a 57-year-old teacher who has had moderately severe neck stiffness and recurrent headache for the past four or five years. No significant previous illness or trauma is reported.

While only periodic pain is experienced, this usually follows strenuous activity and is relieved with rest. Localization of pain, when present, is at the base of the neck with radiation into the shoulder and, on occasion, extending down the arm. No paresthesias are noted.

The head is not carried forward in relationship to the shoulders, but measurable loss (20 to 25 percent) in range of motion is demonstrated. Neurological evaluation and laboratory testing are unremarkable.

In the hyperextension view of John's cervical spine (Fig. 4.11A) a marked hypomobility of cervical rhythm is noted be-low C3. Mobility of the head on the neck above this level is adequate. Note the normal closure of the atlantooccipital interspace. A moderate discogenic spondylosis is noted between C5 and C6 with contiguous osteophytic spur formation noted at the posterior margins. This finding explains the transient pain radiation into the shoulder and arm via neurovascular entrapment or compromise. The remainder of the intervertebral discs are reasonably well maintained, as are the posterior articulating structures.

There is extensive, indeed exuberant, calcifications along the anterior spinal structures from C3 through C7. Can you identify this clinical entity? What must you differentiate this condition from? Are there contraindications to manipulation?

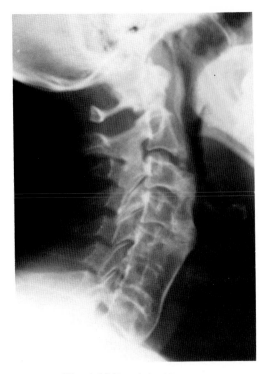

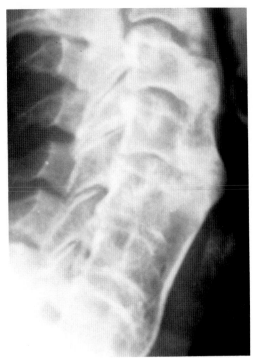

Fig. 4.11B. John W.   **Fig. 4.11C.** John W.

The exuberant calcification with ankylosis of the anterior paraspinal structures is characteristic of *ankylosing hyperostosis* or *Forestier's disease*. At this stage of development, little problem of differentiation from ankylosing spondylitis or discogenic spondylosis is likely. In the early phase it may be tricky.

Forestier's disease is more common in men after the age of 50. The formation of new bone within the anterior soft tissues forms hypertrophic bridges with extensive ankylosis. These bridges do not arise from the vertebral margins, as do osteophytic spur formations, but rather develop in the anterior longitudinal ligaments. Discal thinning is not characteristic. This helps to differentiate the condition from discogenic spondylosis. The age of onset, lack of characteristic sacroiliac and zygapophyseal involvement, and the extensive hypertrophic bridging differentiate this condition from the "bamboo spine" syndesmophytic formations characteristic of ankylosing spondylitis (7, 10).

A radiolucent streaking is often seen between the hyperostotic formations and the vertebral margins, thus ruling out their vertebral origin. The anterior margins of the vertebrae are usually well defined. When ankylosing hyperostosis is found outside of the cervical region, it has been referred to as diffuse idiopathic skeletal hyperostosis or DISH disease. It is probable that both conditions are identical except for the area of involvement.

In John's case a four-year time lapse between Fig. 4.11A and Fig. 4.11, B and C, has occurred. Note the progression in amount and degree of involvement. Due to general hypomobility and the formation of pseudoarthrosis resulting from the extensive hyperostosis, these patients are predisposed to pathological fracture. Accordingly, manipulation is limited to only those areas which do not demonstrate with ankylosis.

Case 4.12

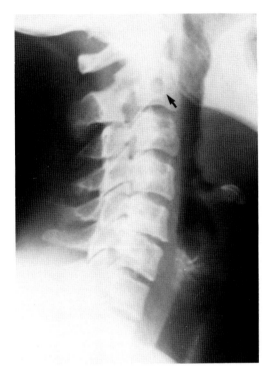

Fig. 4.12. Lori F.

The *degenerative disc disease* between C5 and C6 (Fig. 4.12) is characteristic, with decrease in height of the intervertebral disc and marginal sclerosis. No significant contiguous arthrosis or osteophytosis is as yet demonstrated. This finding, while definitive evidence of impending discogenic spondylosis, nonetheless is of clinical importance due to its decreased interosseous spacing subluxation with attending interarticular facet imbrication. Synovial insult or irritation would be suspect. Alteration of the attending intervertebral foramina would be anticipated with possible neurovascular entrapment.

The *arrow* in Fig. 4.12 is directed towards a circular radiolucency near the centrum of the C2 vertebral body. We are seeing the *foramen transversarium* viewed en face. This is noted frequently at the level of C2 due to its anatomical location and direction coupled with the divergency of the radiographic beam. It represents a normal finding.

Vertebral canal stenosis and the radiculomyelopathic compression syndrome are terms which have crept into the literature with increasing frequency over the past ten years or so. Perhaps most important to recognition of these conditions has been the contribution of transaxial tomography and CT scanning. Prior to the sophistication of these procedures, plain film radiographic findings necessitated myelographic examination for verification. A lack of enthusiasm on the part of the investigator and cooperation by the patients delayed adequate and thorough research. The existence of these conditions and their clinical importance has been known for years, so they cannot be referred to as new entities. Indeed, E. A. Rich, D.C., described a "pedicogenic" stenosis as the etiological source of some L5-S1 discopathy with resultant discogenic spondylosis some 30+ years ago.

While we shall not delve deeply into the subject in this text (there are many excellent papers now available elsewhere (5, 6)), it is proper that a synopsis be included. The plain film radiograph when coupled with clinical findings will still provide evidence of this entity—if you are aware of it.

Stenosis or narrowing of the vertebral canal is developmental or acquired. It may occur at any level but typically is of clinical concern when involving the cervical or lumbosacral regions. Our discussion will deal primarily with the cervical region but bear in mind that similar variations occur at any level.

Developmental stenosis as a pure condition is rather unusual. Symptom patterns associated with it are usually minimal until the situation is altered by the development of spondylotic changes or trauma. With reduction of available canal space, what might be an insignificant lesion in a normal canal can become productive of symptoms of a myelopathic, radicular or combined nature.

The acquired stenosis is common. Any condition which results in narrowing of the canal and its recesses, causes intrusion, compression and functional disturbance at that level of the cord. The resulting symptom pattern may be local but is most commonly seen to present with widely varying patterns, dependent upon the cord tract or vascular structure involved. The most prominent level of involvement is at the C5 or C6 level. This may produce myelopathic symptoms, such as weakness of the arms and hands, a staggering, wide gait, and interosseous muscular atrophy of the hands. This instability in walking has been likened to "walking like a drunk." Duration of symptoms varies from weeks to years. With extension of intrusion into the lateral recesses and the intervertebral foramina, shoulder and arm pain appears, but this can be quite variable, intermittent and inconstant.

Developmental stenosis may be asymptomatic for a long time, but in the event of discal herniation or spondylotic change, otherwise minimal lesions become highly important. Acquired stenotic lesions are mainly those of middle age but have been seen in younger age groups as well as in the elderly.

While the list of etiological agents capable of producing vertebral canal stenosis varies from retrolisthesis to Paget's disease, from trauma to spondylosis, the awareness that symptom expression may result at some distance peripheral to the site of stenosis should accentuate your interest and concern.

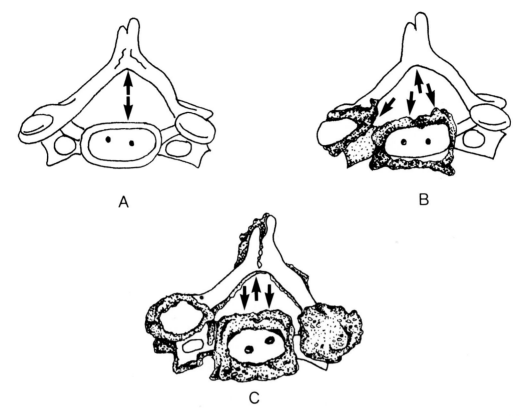

Fig. 4.13. *A*: Schematic of normal C6 vertebra. *Arrows* indicate the normal sagittal measurement taken from the posterior vertebral margin to the spinous process-laminae junction. Note the wide lateral recesses and wide, smooth foraminal canals. *B*: Spondylotic changes have produced stenosis or narrowing of the vertebral canal with decrease of the sagittal diameter. The lateral recess on the left and the foraminal canals are intruded upon by osteophytic spurs of the articular facet and covertebral joints of Luschka. Note obstruction and obliteration of the foramen transversarium. *C*: Gross spondylotic changes of the articular facets, mostly on the right, as well as the posterior vertebral margin. Compression and stenosis of the spinal canal, foraminal canals and vascular foramen (5).

In Fig. 4.13*A* the *arrows* indicate the normal floor-to-ceiling *measurement of the vertebral canal.* This measurement is made by measuring between the posterior surface of the vertebral body to the nearest edge of the fused portion of the spinous process. This will provide the sagittal diameter of the vertebral canal. In Fig. 4.13*B* can be seen the funnel-shaped appearance of the canal. The normal canal is about 13 mm. Values below this are significant, and those above 15 mm are regarded as normal (4, 5). It must be pointed out that when intrusions into the canal are evident, i.e., spondylosis, the measurement is taken between its posterior margin and not from the originating vertebral body. This provides the functional use of this measurement (Fig. 4.14).

In Fig. 4.13, *B* and *C* are schematic representations of various changes to the vertebral canal, lateral recesses, posterior articular facets, vascular canal and foramen transversarium—all having produced

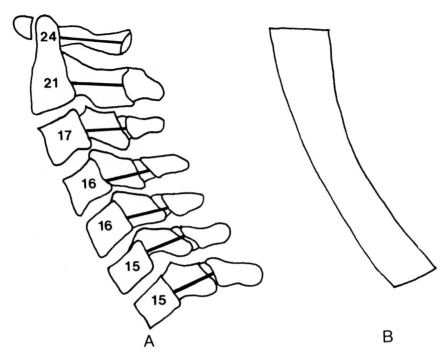

Fig. 4.14. *A*: Schematic demonstrating the normal sagittal measurement of the spinal canal. The measurement is taken from the posterior aspect of the vertebral body, or spondylotic intrusion, to the spinous process-laminae junction. *B*: Line tracing of the spinal canal size and shape in *A* (4).

some form of compression or stenosis to normal interspace. The exceptions to this are those osteophytic spurs located on the anterior surface of the vertebral body. The location of bony overgrowths are significant if the ridges and spurs from the central and neural arches are productive of neural compressive changes. In addition to the spondylotic intrusion, other compres-

sive agents include a thickened yellow ligament and discal herniation. While emphasis is placed on osseous overgrowth, it should be recalled that cartilaginous and fibrotic changes are of equal significance. Intrusions capable of producing cord and nerve root compression as well as vascular impairment are most likely to occur in hyperextension (5, 6).

Case 4.13

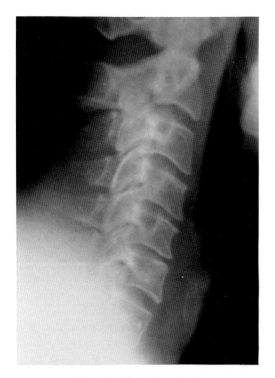

Fig. 4.15A. Dennis A.

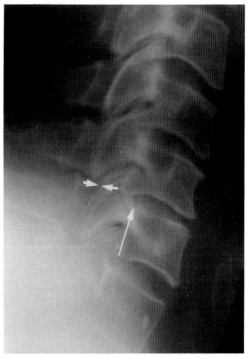

Fig. 4.15B. Dennis A.

Dennis is a 32-year-old man who has had periodic stiffness of his lower neck for some time. It has worsened in the past two years since a rear end auto collision. Over the last six months he began to experience transient pain and numbness over the peripheral course of the radial nerve. He can produce the neuropathic pattern at will by mere hyperextension of the head and neck.

Chiropractic manipulation was employed over the last four months with only temporary, partial relief.

The patient has moderate thinning of the C5–C6 intervertebral disc. No evidence of contiguous arthrosis is noted, however, suggesting hypoplasia vis à vis degeneration. Anatomical variance in the AP measurement of C6 and C7 as compared to those vertebral bodies above is seen. This variance has created a "kink" or narrowing in the vertebral canal due to partial stenosis (*double arrows* in Fig. 4.15F).

While the radiculomyelopathic compression syndrome is typically due to osteophytic intrusion, any condition which produces stenosis is capable of inducing a similar clinical picture. In this case the degree of *developmental stenosis* was apparently tolerated even in the presence of anatomical instability, until trauma induced thickening by cicatricial fibrosis and/or hypertrophy of the yellow ligament. This additional crowding of the vertebral canal has precipitated radicular compression, particularly in hyperextension.

For the purposes of this text we would like to point out a few of the more salient features of, and between, rheumatoid arthritis and ankylosing spondylitis. Both conditions present with similar pathogenesis and affect synovial joints. *Rheumatoid arthritis* is generally considered a condition involving the peripheral joints, i.e., the hand, wrist and foot. The cervical spine is frequently affected, but the sacroiliac joints are only occasionally involved. It often begins during adolescence, more often during the third decade, and the most serious incidence is two to three times greater in females.

In *ankylosing spondylitis* the age incidence is about the same as rheumatoid arthritis but occurs 10 to 15 times more frequently in males. Typically it begins in the lower lumbar spine or sacroiliac joints and ascends the spine. The condition is predominately one of spinal involvement. Its comparative clinical frequency is approximately one-fifth that of rheumatoid arthritis.

As the pathogenesis is similar, most older texts refer to ankylosing spondylitis as rheumatoid arthritis of the spine, i.e., rheumatoid spondylitis. It is also referred to as Marie-Strümpell disease. Clinically, rheumatoid arthritis and ankylosing spondylitis are quite dissimilar.

In both conditions the joints of involvement begin with thickening and swelling of the synovium. The thickened synovium undergoes a chronic exudative inflammatory reaction. Thereafter, progression of the disease produces hyperplasia, fibrin formation and resultant granulation tissue, i.e., pannus formation. This pannus formation within the joint releases lytic enzymes which cause cartilage fragmentation with eventual subchondral cystic absorption of the articular plate. Eventually the entire joint space is filled with thickened synovium and granular pannus. The articular plate is destroyed and the joint distorted. Fibrous adhesion formations then occur from one subchondral area to another, producing fibrous ankylosis. Eventually calcification followed by ossification of the fibrotic adhesions occurs to produce a bony or osseous ankylosis, with resultant loss of joint function (1, 18).

It is well to remember that the above description applies to synovial joints. In so doing you will recall that in the spine this would restrict involvement to the posterior articulating facets, the atlantoodontoid interspaces, and costovertebral articulations. In ankylosing spondylitis, calcification of the paraspinous ligaments occurs, providing the "eggshell" appearance surrounding and between the vertebrae, resulting in a fixed ankylosed spine, i.e., the "bamboo spine" or "poker spine." Prior to total fixation by this paraspinal calcification, the corners of the vertebral bodies give rise to the typical paravertebral ossifications known as syndesmophytes. The syndesmophytes develop in the region of the vertebral body erosions and anulus fibrosus and extend vertically (as opposed to the horizontal direction of osteophytes), bridging the adjacent intervertebral disc space. While they appear delicate originally, as thickening occurs they become well defined and are most responsible for the "bamboo" appearance of the well-advanced case of ankylosing spondylitis.

Osteoporosis is common to both rheumatoid arthritis and ankylosing spondylitis. Deep erosion or cyst-like lesions are frequent in rheumatoid arthritis but uncommon to ankylosing spondylitis. The bone erosions of ankylosing spondylitis are usually superficial and associated with reactive sclerosis, often producing a "fluffy" appearance, particularly at the ischial and femoral trochanteric margins (22).

Atlantoaxial subluxation, the result of synovium involvement, is frequently observed in rheumatoid arthritis. Indeed, should the anterior atlantodental interval (ADI) exceed 3 mm, consideration of rheumatoid arthritis as an etiological source is mandated (20).

In the advanced stage of either disease the potential for pathological fracture as a complication of the osteoporotic ankylosed spine is of prime concern. Manipulation must be performed with caution.

Case 4.14

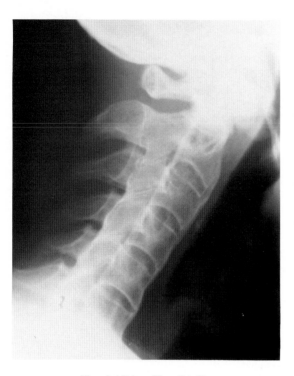

Fig. 4.16A. Timothy E.

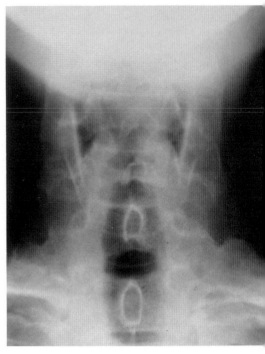

Fig. 4.16B. Timothy E.

Fig. 4.16 shows *ankylosing spondylitis* in a 40-year-old man, demonstrating total fusion or ankylosis of the zygapophyseal articulations. Note the characteristic "eggshell" calcification extending along the anterior spine. The AP radiograph shows the extent of lateral joint involvement and the "bamboo spine" appearance. The intervertebral discs appear reasonably well maintained, and no evidence of concurrent degenerative spondylosis is seen. The anterior ADI is not involved. The at-lantooccipital rhythm has been maintained, and nodding of the head permitted. This later finding is not unusual due to the lack of posterior joints and ankylosis at this level. Total loss of interbody joint mobility has occurred below C2, the result of ankylosis.

Fig. 4.16A was taken with the patient in a neutral lateral position yet shows marked forward displacement of the head and neck. This posture is quite characteristic, clinically.

Case 4.15

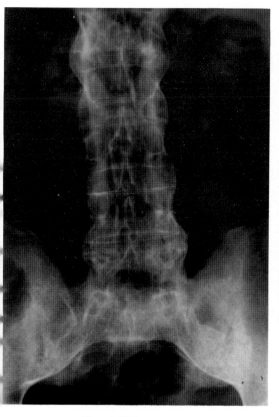

Fig. 4.17A. Mark A.

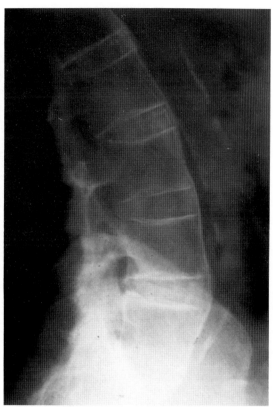

Fig. 4.17B. Mark A.

Mark is a 54-year-old man with a long-standing history of spinal immobility. While his neck has escaped involvement, the thoracic and lumbar spine and pelvis are all involved. The normal spinal curves have been preserved except for a minimal thoracic kyphosis. On observation, the act of walking and flexion of the spine appears to occur entirely from the hips. The forward displacement of the head and neck in relation to the trunk, frequently seen in these cases, is not applicable in Mark's case.

Historically, Mark developed moderate pain with stiffness of his lumbosacral and sacroiliac joints at the age of 22. A rather stormy clinical course followed over the next ten years, with various forms of treatment attempted. None provided abatement of symptom expression or halted progress of involvement. Fortunately, the past ten years or so has seen a decrease in pain. The remaining stiffness and lack of mobility has of course hampered his way of life.

There is said to be a greater incidence of cardiac involvement in this condition than in rheumatoid arthritis (11). This complication is more apt to involve the aortic valve, its ring and the ascending aortic segment. In Mark, the degree of atherosclerotic plaqueing seen in the descending aorta and iliac arteries (Fig. 4.17B) may be related to the condition but is probably coincidental.

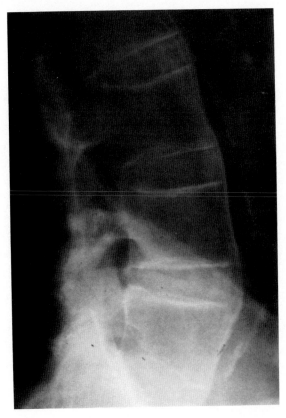

Fig. 4.17 C.   Mark A.

Mark demonstrates with a classical case of *ankylosing spondylitis*.

You will note in Fig. 4.17A the characteristic "bamboo" appearance at the L1–L2 level. The remaining levels all have varying degrees of this paraspinal ligamentous calcification. Characteristically, the thoracolumbar region is the first to demonstrate the "bamboo" appearance.

The sacroiliac joints are markedly obliterated, with irregular margination and patchy sclerosis seen. Anklylosis is near complete on the right. Interestingly, when ankylosis is complete, the patchy marginal sclerosis will disappear, indicating the lack of stress to the completely fused bone.

In Fig. 4.17, *B* and *C*, is seen the typical squared off appearance of the anterior vertebral bodies. Calcification and ossification of the anterior soft tissues and anterior longitudinal ligament are well seen. Note the bulging of the intervertebral discs which thus far have maintained their normal height. While not adequately demonstrated in these pictures, fusion of the posterior articulating facets is near complete.

The degree of osteoporosis noted throughout the study is quite typical. Pathological fractures are often encountered with minimal stress due to the osteoporosis and immobility of the spine. Manipulation must therefore be done with great caution.

Case 4.16

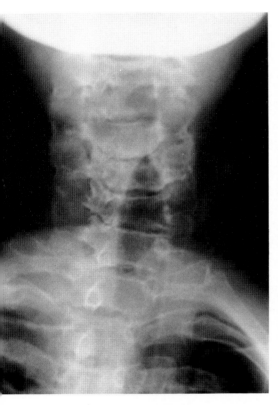

Fig. 4.18A. Pamela T.

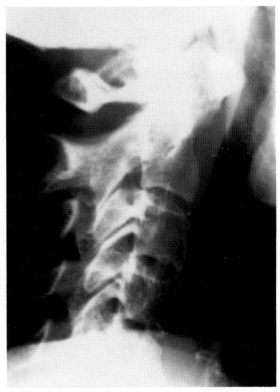

Fig. 4.18B. Pamela T.

Pamela is 52-year-old insurance secretary who has had chronic ache and pain of her peripheral joints and neck for many years. Following what was considered a minor "fender bender," rather severe symptoms of throbbing headache, numbness and tingling of both upper extremities, and transient nausea began. She also reports feeling "weird" all over, including a heaviness of her lower extremities with difficulty in walking.

Examination indicates diminished neurological and deep tendon reflexes and loss of tensile and grip strength. Tactile sensation is intact. There is a diminution in range of motion of the head and neck in all ranges but negative neck compression testing. Fusiform swelling is noted of the interphalangeal joints of both hands.

Careful review of Fig. 4.18, A and B, will indicate several concurrent conditions and with the history provide an explanation of complaints. Be careful. It is well to remember that quite frequently a patient will present with more than one condition at a time.

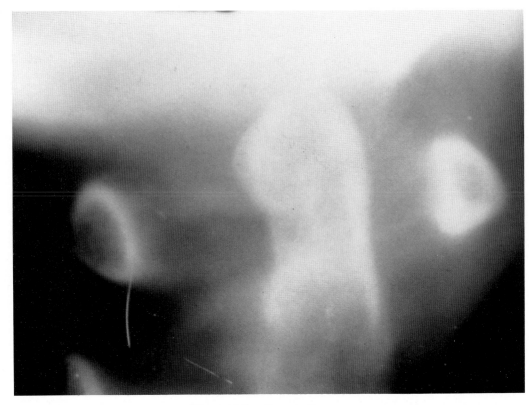

Fig. 4.18C. Pamela T.

The lateral wedging of the lower cervical segments is obvious. While discal thinning is seen, the most obvious alteration is *covertebral joints of Luschka arthrosis* on the left. Vertebral artery compromise would be suspect. Examination of the lateral view indicates reasonably well maintained intervertebral discs as visualized. The zygapophyseal articulations are intact. The presence of a *ponticulus posticus* is noted of the C1 posterior arch and is considered of little clinical importance.

Careful review of the lateral film indicates a marked increase of the anterior atlantodental interval (ADI). In Fig. 4.18C, a tomogram of C1 demonstrates this marked increase of the ADI. This finding should suggest anterior displacement of C1 on C2, the result of increased width of the synovium due to inflammation, or the loss of ligamentous restraint following tearing of the transverse ligament. In this case the symptom complex, which includes interphalangeal fusiform swelling, is confirmatory evidence that the increased ADI is the result of *rheumatoid arthritis*. As mentioned earlier, an increase of the ADI of over 3 mm should always cause suspicion of rheumatoid arthritis as an etiological agent.

With the anterior displacement of C1 on C2 a narrowing or *stenosis of the vertebral canal* occurs. In this case the stenosis developed gradually and cord adaptation was permitted. The addition of acute trauma, however, was sufficient to produce a cord concussion with transient nervous system shock. This explains the onset of CNS symptomatology. Fortunately, no permanent sequelae occurred.

Case 4.17

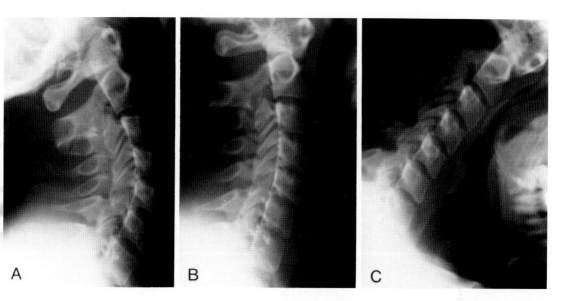

Fig. 4.19, *A*, *B* and *C*.   Laura L.

Laura is a 23-year-old woman who had been involved in an automobile accident, striking her head against the windshield, two days prior to this examination. She had been seen at the hospital trauma room, radiographed, told she had no fracture, provided a cervical collar and instructed to rest for a week. Her minor strain should then be better.

She has experienced headache, nausea, vertigo and transient blurred vision since. The neck is quite tender and when rotating her head to either side she reports aggravation of complaints.

Examination reveals positive head-neck compression testing. Range of motion examination is markedly limited throughout. Palpable tenderness is found at the suboccipital region, and moderate paraspinal muscular splinting is noted throughout, with extension into the right trapezius. During the radiographic examination, hyperflexion positioning produced transient aggravation of vertigo and pain.

After careful review of Fig. 4.19, *A*, *B* and *C*, your diagnosis should be easy. The AP and oblique views are noncontributory. What treatment do you feel will most benefit this patient? Is manipulation required on a frequent basis? Also, the patient asks how soon she can return to active sports activity—any restrictions?

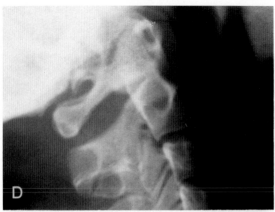

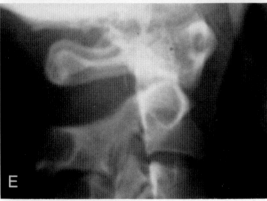

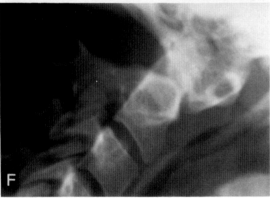

Figs. 4.19, *D, E* and *F.* Laura L.

In the discussion of rheumatoid arthritis we stressed the importance and significance of the anterior atlantodental interval (ADI). This case highlights the importance of this finding, albeit of a traumatic origin.

You may recall that the increase of over 3 mm was of importance. In disease it is caused by an increase in size of the intervening synovium (between the odontoid and the anterior tubercle of C1) (18, 20). This causes forward displacement of C1, stretching of the transverse ligament (which forms the sling behind the odontoid to restrict anterior movement of C1 on C2), and the propensity towards vertebral canal stenosis with or without cord compression.

In Laura's case a traumatic *rupture or tear of the transverse ligament* with hypermobility of C1 on C2 is obvious by extrapolation. Notice in the neutral and flexion views the increased ADI. In the extension view, complete loss of the ADI is seen. The odontoid process now serves to prevent posterior excursion of C1 on C2. The anterior movement of C1 is graphic in Fig. 4.19, *E* and *F*. With it, attending decrease of the vertebral canal measurement has occurred. Cord compression, by symptom review, is not severe.

Healing will depend basically on cicatricial fibrosis (adhesion formation) which, hopefully, will stabilize the segment(s). Manipulation should be performed sparingly initially, if at all, so that fixation might occur. Care should be given to appropriate postural habits, including those during sleep, via some form of stabilization. Laura's activities in the gym are to be totally restricted for six months, when reevaluation will be done.

Case 4.18

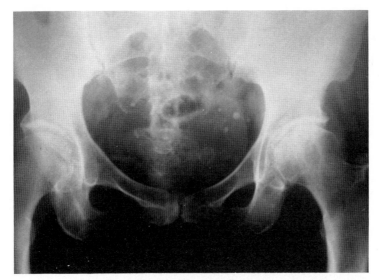

Fig. 4.20A. Florence D.

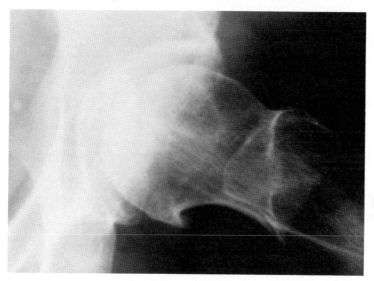

Fig. 4.20B. Florence D.

Florence is a 63-year-old Caucasian woman who has developed chronic, recurrent pain in the right hip region over the past few years. It has become increasingly difficult for her to walk or stand for prolonged periods.

While Florence reports that the combination of heat and rest relieves the pain and stiffness, the relief is short-lived. About one month ago she began to feel that her hip would "go out" on her at any moment. A noticeable limp has appeared, in response to pain.

Examination indicates no neurological deficit, and orthopedic testing, including Patrick's fabere test, indicates the complaint to be localized to the right hip joint itself. There is no evidence of muscular atrophy. While minimal joint effusion is suspect, it is not adequately demonstrated or defined.

The radiograph (Fig. 4.20A) is near conclusive. Can you identify and diagnose the condition? What is the best descriptive term for the condition? Is it progressive; can it be substantially altered from the change(s) now present? What is the overall prognosis? Will any biomechanical alterations ensue in other parts of the body as a result of this condition?

125

Florence is suffering with a moderately early case of *degenerative joint disease (DJD)* involving the right hip. While progression of the condition is the rule, treatment aimed at restoration or revitalization of the vascular flow is often helpful in reducing the rate of progress. The pain in DJD is often the result of synovial irritation and inflammation. Programmed non-weight-bearing exercises and instruction in avoidance of activities causing capsular fatigue or stress are often helpful. Should the degenerative breakdown continue unabated, it is probable that surgical intervention with total hip replacement will eventually be recommended. Due to the altered weight bearing, both prior and subsequent to any surgical repair, excessive stress can be anticipated to the lumbopelvic spine. Biomechanical alterations may be anticipated which will require attention of their own.

Selection of this case was intentional. The radiographic changes, while consistent and obvious to the well-trained eye, are nonetheless somewhat vague. Please don't get upset if you missed it. As we continue over the next page or two you will increase that awareness necessary to retrospectively define it with confidence. It is true that hindsight is always 20–20!

Because man is an upright biped, he is necessarily subject to the convenience *and* stress of weight bearing. Without venturing into a discussion of the various forms of stress, e.g., weight, posture, hormonal, emotions, etc., may I simply state that the term degenerative is particularly apropos and is the result of stress and aging.

Formerly referred to as osteoarthritis, a rather all-inclusive term, DJD is best understood if its use is confined to the peripheral joints of the appendicular skeleton. It has a predilection for the interphalangeal joints of the hands, particularly the terminal ones, and the weight-bearing joints, such as the hip and knee. Secondary DJD may occur in any joint altered by disease or trauma. It may be a sequel to arthrodesis of an adjacent joint and is often seen in the ankles and feet of athletes (1, 18). While the changes are the same when affecting the spine, these areas have select terms of their own; e.g., DJD of the covertebral joints of Luschka is best known as covertebral joints of Luschka arthrosis.

Case 4.19

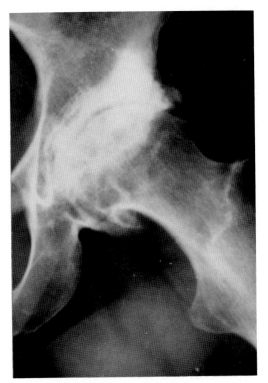

Fig. 4.20C. Arthur C.

Degenerative joint disease begins radiographically with a nonuniform narrowing of the cartilaginous interarticular joint space. It may be uniform when cartilage destruction is advanced. This cartilaginous breakdown evokes a reparative response in an attempt at remodeling. Subchondral sclerosis and cyst-like radiolucencies develop. These cyst-like areas have a thin rim of sclerosis and rarely interrupt cortical continuity. Cartilage hyperplasia occurs at the joint margins which undergo new bone production with resultant osteophytic formations. Osteoporosis may develop, but this is less characteristic in DJD than in rheumatoid arthritis. In DJD it is usually the result of disuse.

In some severe long-standing cases of DJD of weight-bearing joints, subchondral destruction may occur, producing deformity. Occasionally, bony ankylosis may develop and must not be misinterpreted as evidence of rheumatoid, psoriatic or prior infectious arthritis.

In summation, DJD is characterized by narrowing of the interarticular joint space, subchondral sclerosis with cyst-like radiolucencies, and marginal osteophytosis. The overall picture is one of the body's response to stress in an attempt at repair. It is the most common of all the arthritides (1, 18).

Case 4.20

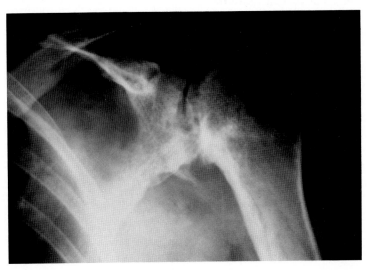

Fig. 4.20D. Karl A.

Fig. 4.20*A* and 4.20*B* demonstrate uneven narrowing of the interarticular joint space of the right hip. Comparison evaluation with the left side may be necessary. Moderate subchondral sclerosis is seen, and small cyst-like radiolucencies are noted. One rather large cyst-like area is seen within the centrum of the femoral head, best seen in Fig. 4.20*B*. Note the thin rim of sclerosis. This case, as mentioned, is moderately early DJD.

Fig. 4.20*C* shows a severe case of DJD involving the right hip. Note the extensive osteophytic spurring at both superior and inferior acetabular margins. The cyst-like areas of radiolucency are well visualized. Extensive subchondral sclerosis of the acetabular roof is present. The narrowing of the joint space is marked, suggesting probably immobility. Arthur subsequently underwent surgical arthrodesis of the right hip with good results.

Fig. 4.20*D* shows a severe DJD of the left shoulder. Because the left shoulder is a non-weight-bearing joint, you might wonder about this—and rightfully so. DJD is not as commonly involved in this joint because it is non-weight-bearing. However, in Karl's case the etiology is posttraumatic. Extensive cartilaginous destruction occurred with disruption of blood flow. The development of DJD was a sequel. You will note the radiolucent fracture line still remaining in the humeral shaft. Osteoporosis is present throughout the humeral head, accounting for the poor radiographic visualization.

Case 4.21

Fig. 4.20*E* shows minimal DJD but is included here to check your present comprehension. Remember 20–20 hindsight? Notice the uneven narrowing of the joint space. Small cyst-like areas are developing in the subchondral region of the humeral head. Remember that this joint is non-weight-bearing, and thus the reactive sclerosis will be less intense and slower to appear. None is present as yet.

Notice the arrowhead configuration of *synovial chondrometaplasia* (1) located immediately below the glenoid-humeral interspace, within the soft tissue (*arrow* on Fig. 4.20*E*). This represents a free fragment of cartilage which resulted from the same injury that produced the fracture seen extending from the humeral neck, running diagonally into the shaft. You did see that, didn't you? Of course you did!

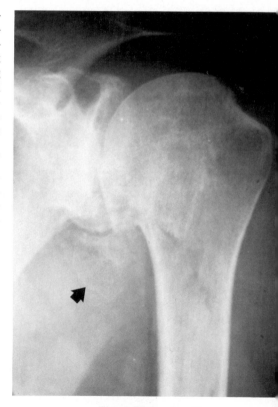

Fig. 4.20E.   Ina M.

Section 5

Benign Variations

Case 5.1

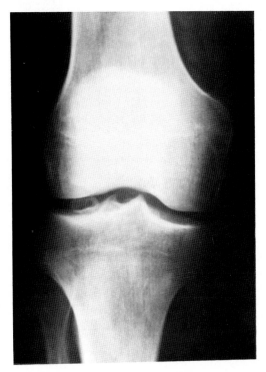

Fig. 5.1 A. Bo J.

Bo is a 20-year-old man who has been bothered by transient knee pain, following severe exercise, for two or three years. Each time his knee has "locked" on him, it would ease off in a matter of minutes, and only residual tenderness would remain for several days. His coach told him it was muscle spasms and not to worry about it.

The past few weeks have been preseason basketball practice, and Bo has experienced near-constant knee pain. The knee is locking more frequently, and the pain is more intense.

On examination the posterior popliteal fossa is "mushy" with some edema. No significant hyperemia is noted. Reflexes are maintained. No evidence of meniscal tearing or ligamentous laxity is noted.

Fig. 5.1A indicates a probable "joint mouse" within the lateral interarticular joint space. Careful review suggests others as well. The area of calcification does not coincide with a juxta-articular defect of similar size and shape, so often found in osteochondrosis dissecans.

What conditions are most frequently the cause of loose bodies or a "joint mouse" in an articulation? What joints are most frequently involved? Is surgery always necessary? What type of tissue is most commonly involved?

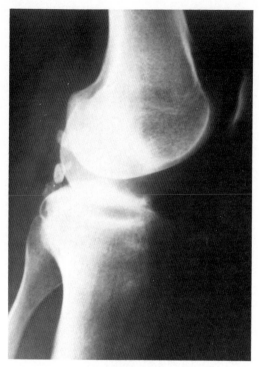

Fig. 5.1 _B_.   Bo J.

The lateral radiograph (Fig. 5.1B) demonstrates not one loose body, but several. Close observation will reveal both calcification and ossification. This is not unusual in a case of _osteochondromatosis_.

Generally initiated by trauma, this condition is most often seen in young and middle-aged adults. It typically follows the sequence of posttraumatic synovitis, synovial hypertrophy which forms cartilaginous masses, followed by calcification or ossification with resultant irregular ovoid or circular radiodensities which occupy the joint space. A laminated appearance is common in the larger formation. The growth in size of these joint bodies is made possible in that they derive their nutriment from the surrounding synovial fluid (19, 22).

While contained within the joint capsule, these loose bodies do not pose a threat to joint function until migrating between joint surfaces. At that time the "locking" of the joint is common. If these locking bodies are not surgically removed a chronic synovitis with joint effusion will occur and predispose towards degenerative joint disease. Those which are confined within the joint capsule but do not enter between the joint surfaces may lie dormant for long periods of time or until trauma intercedes to prompt an acute synovitis.

Osteochondromatosis is most frequently seen in the knee but occasionally may be found in the elbow or hip.

It is well to note that loose bodies or "joint mice" are most commonly associated with osteochondrosis dissecans, osteochondromatosis, interarticular fracture with separation of a fragment of cartilage, meniscal fragmentation in the knee, and degenerative joint disease.

Case 5.2

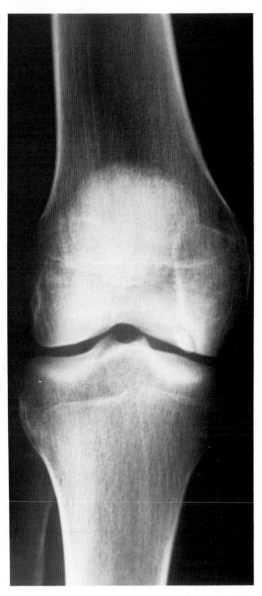

Fig. 5.2 A.   Wilson W.

Wilson is a 16-year-old boy and local high school basketball standout. His talent "off the boards" has grown each season to the point that his future seems to pivot around his physical ability.

For some time now Wilson has had constant pain and discomfort of the right knee. While he hasn't had any "locking of the knee, the constant repetition of rebounding has caused exacerbation of pain and moderate swelling to occur.

As with most serious athletes, Wilson has been willing to "grin and bear it," until recently. He has become concerned now because the pain and swelling do not abate as quickly as they once did following the use of ice packs.

Physical examination was inconclusive except to demonstrate that all ligaments appear intact. Fig. 5.2A is definitive, with little doubt left as to the diagnosis. Can you spot the problem and attach the correct diagnostic term? What advice as to treatment will you offer Wilson? Is it the same advice you would offer a nonathelete?

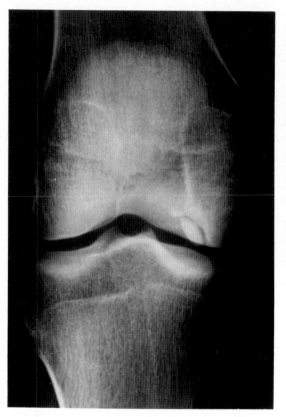

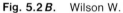

Fig. 5.2 B. Wilson W.

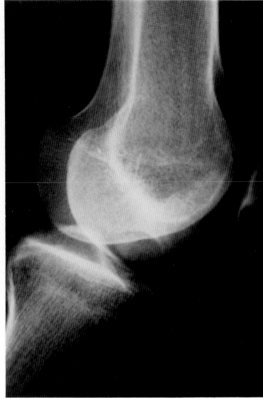

Fig. 5.2 C. Wilson W.

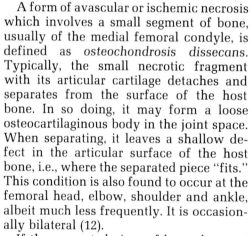

A form of avascular or ischemic necrosis which involves a small segment of bone, usually of the medial femoral condyle, is defined as *osteochondrosis dissecans*. Typically, the small necrotic fragment with its articular cartilage detaches and separates from the surface of the host bone. In so doing, it may form a loose osteocartilaginous body in the joint space. When separating, it leaves a shallow defect in the articular surface of the host bone, i.e., where the separated piece "fits." This condition is also found to occur at the femoral head, elbow, shoulder and ankle, albeit much less frequently. It is occasionally bilateral (12).

If the separated piece of bone does not become completely separated, it may remain within its cavity either becoming absorbed or eventually developing a new blood supply and undergoing revitalization (1). This process dictates avoidance of reinjury, and much time.

In Wilson's case the fragment had separated yet was contained. If he had been willing to assume a sedentary life-style, he would have been a candidate for absorption or revitalization. However, he was anxious to "get on with it," so surgical intervention was elected. Removal of the fragment was done, and he was returned to active participation in basketball. He's not in the pros—yet!

Case 5.3

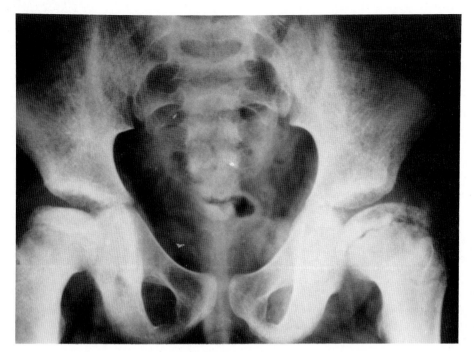

Fig. 5.3 A.   Donny T.

Donny is a 9-year-old boy who presented for examination due to a noticeable painless limp. While unsure of the exact onset, his mother relates that about four months ago Donny hurt his right hip during a "rocket" football game. At the time, slight swelling had been noted. With a few days of rest the swelling and pain had abated. The football season was over, and no further incident of trauma could be recalled. His limp had developed gradually over the past six to eight weeks.

The examination indicated joint tension and moderate tenderness to palpation of the entire right hip. No evidence of joint effusion, neurological deficit or muscular atrophy was demonstrated. When walking, the patient seemed to "throw his right hip" in an arc-like fashion, with resultant noticeable limp. No pain was reported.

With the history provided, would you conclude that Donny has a transient synovitis of the right hip, or would you anticipate a more complex problem? Why? Fig. 5.3A indicates what clinical entity? Can you estimate the stage of involvement, and are there any ancillary treatment procedures which you would employ?

First examination of Fig. 5.3A demonstrates lateral displacement of the head of the right femur. This is due to hyperemia of the synovium and is a frequent finding in acute transient synovitis as well as in the present condition. The history precludes an acute transient synovitis in that, as the name implies, the time lapse between injury and presentation is too great. Also a limp, if present, is definitely not painless in acute transient synovitis (23).

Comparison of the right and left femoral epiphysis indicates a definite flattening on the right. In Fig. 5.3B, areas of cystic formation and textural abnormalities are seen. Fragmentation, a classic finding, is noted of the lateral half of the capital femoral epiphysis.

The combination of lateral displacement, diminution in size with flattening, cystic formations with textural alteration, fragmentation of the capital femoral epiphysis, and clinical presentation of a painless limp are classical manifestations of osteochondrosis or ischemic necrosis, perhaps best known as *Legg-Calvé-Perthes disease* (1, 23).

In Donny's case the degree of fragmentation and flattening can be expected to worsen. As the alteration of the epiphysis is due to avascular or ischemic necrosis, a greater degree of bone death within the epiphysis is anticipated due to lack of blood supply. Once the active phase of destruction ceases, a reparative and reconstruction stage(s) appears. The end result will be a femoral head which is markedly flattened with widening of the femoral neck—the so-called "mushroom" deformity. A widened interarticular joint space

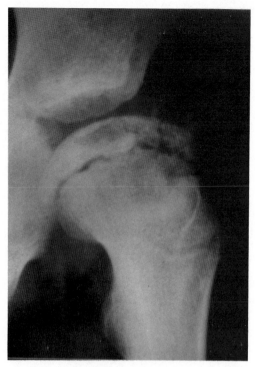

Fig. 5.3 B.   Donny T.

persists late into the disease.

As the condition progresses from destruction (avascularity) to repair (revascularization) and to reconstruction (growth stress), it is not unusual for several years or longer to elapse. In order to lessen the degree of deformity during the destruction and repair phases, it is well to employ some form of sling brace or orthosis which will prevent weight bearing on the affected hip. In addition, measures designed to increase vascularity of the involved structures is advised.

Case 5.4

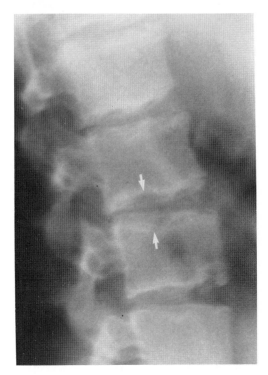

Fig. 5.4.   Robbie M.

Robbie is a 14-year-old boy who is physically more mature than most boys his age. As a result he usually is asked to do the jobs typically reserved for "older kids."

After helping work on his dad's car engine over the past two weeks, during which time he was asked to support or hold heavy loads while draped over the car's fender, he developed constant pain and discomfort in the lower thoracic and upper lumbar regions. The pain was relieved by rest but reappeared soon after becoming weight bearing.

Examination revealed bilateral paraspinal palpatory tenderness with spasm from T8 through L3. No significant pain radiation was noted. Percussion testing was moderately positive. No other neurological, orthopedic or laboratory tests were revealing. No significant limitation in range of motion of the thoracolumbar spine was noted, albeit uncomfortable in forward flexion.

In Robbie's case a frequently encountered concurrent condition can be identified (*arrows* in Fig. 5.4)—Schmorl's nodes. You may recall that Schmorl's nodes are the result of intrusion by discal material through a minor end-plate infraction at the remnant site of the notochord. This is considered by some authors to indicate a defect in end-plate ossification and therefore may also suggest an etiological basis for the concurrent condition in Robbie. A note of caution: Schmorl's nodes are far more frequent than the condition under question, and often are found existing alone at all levels of the spine.

Can you identify and name the condition? What is the most frequent age of occurrence, and what, if any, sequelae must be guarded against?

Case 5.5

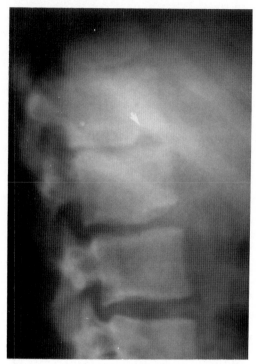

Fig. 5.5. Les T.

Les is a 16-year-old boy who has had periodic lower thoracic pain for the past two years. Because the discomfort was periodic and relieved by rest, he did not seek attention for it until now. Recently, stiffness and ache have become constant, and he is uncomfortable after standing for prolonged periods of time at work.

While this case is more advanced, indeed healed, than that of Robbie's in Fig. 5.4, both are referred to as *Scheuermann's disease* or kyphosis juvenilis.

Representing an osteochondrosis of the vertebral epiphyseal plate, Scheuermann's disease occurs between the ages of 12 and 16. It affects boys and girls equally. The complaint of pain which is relieved by lying down is characteristic. The lower thoracic and upper lumbar spines are involved most frequently. As with all of the osteochondroses, ischemic necrosis is considered a prime etiological agent. Some suggest, however, that similar to the Schmorl's node development, it may represent mere faulty ossification of the vertebral epiphysis (23).

In the early phase the epiphyseal plates or secondary ossification centers become irregular and fragmented in their appearance. Occasionally they are somewhat sclerotic. The vertebral body becomes irregular with notching at their anterior margins (see Fig. 5.5). With growth, the vertebral body becomes wedge-shaped with decreases in its height anteriorly (Fig. 5.5). This may proceed to develop a thoracic kyphosis—with no gibbus formation, however. Discal thinning is a frequent localized finding. Once ossification is complete, the deformity of anterior vertebral wedging, thoracic kyphosis, discal thinning and marginal irregularity of the vertebral bodies persist. This frequently leads to secondary degenerative changes with considerable osteophytosis (12).

Case 5.6

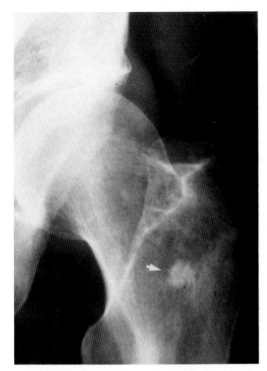

Fig. 5.6 A.   Marty W.

A sometimes confusing finding is well demonstrated in Fig. 5.6, *A* and *B*, of Marty's right proximal femur.

An ill-defined, dense radiopacity is noted, surrounded by normal architecture. No evidence of surrounding reactive scle-rosis, loss or lack of substance, marginal containment or evidence of repair. The cortical, chondral and periosteal markings are normal. No soft-tissue involvement is seen.

This represents an area of *nonreticulated bone* or bone island.

When seen, this finding indicates a lack of trabecular network or pattern through a small island or portion of bone. Thus, the typical bony architecture is lacking. It represents a normal anatomical variant and is rarely, if ever, of clinical importance.

Being within the medullary portion of bone excludes free ossa, loose bodies, "joint mice" and intercalary bone.

Differential consideration must be given to osteopoikilosis and the button sequestrum of osteoblastic metastasis (12). These are typically multiple and well circumscribed. The dense structureless appearance of an enostosis or enostoma may be similar but is larger and denser, tends to progressively enlarge, and generally demonstrates contiguous architectural derangement, i.e., osteoporosis. The osteomas are well-circumscribed and rounded radiopacities (13).

Nonreticulated areas of bone are most commonly found in the proximal femur, distal humerus and pelvis. Its size may vary but seldom is larger than that shown in Fig. 5.6, *A* and *B*.

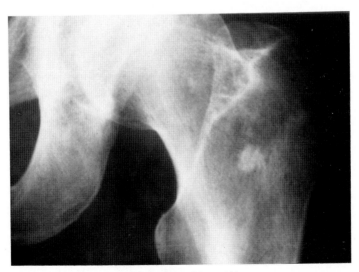

Fig. 5.6 B.   Marty W.

Case 5.7

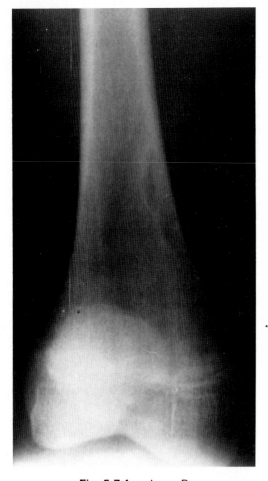

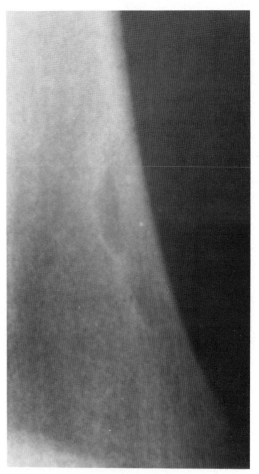

Fig. 5.7 A. Jason P.

Fig. 5.7 B. Jason P.

Jason is an 8-year-old boy who injured his knee while wrestling. Radiographic examination (Fig. 5.7) uncovered a relatively common abnormality as an incidental finding.

A rather large number of normal children demonstrate with one or more of these lesions, known as a *fibrous cortical defect*. Usually discovered between the ages of four and eight, the lesion is more often found in males than in females and is asymptomatic.

The lesions are typically small ovoid, round, or flame-shaped radiolucencies and demonstrate a shallow cortical defect. Its margins are well defined and are seen as a smooth or scalloped, thin dense line (13).

The most common location is the posterior medial aspect of the distal femoral metaphysis, followed by the proximal tibia and fibula. Other tubular bones may be involved.

As mentioned, the lesion is asymptomatic and, while indicating a variant of cellular fibrous tissue placement, typically regresses spontaneously with no residual deformity. Once regression is complete, normal appearance of bone occurs. Rarely, a small focus of dense sclerosis remains. In some instances, failure of regression occurs and proliferation ensues. With this proliferation the lesion tends to migrate from the metaphysis towards the diaphysis. Found again incidentally, between the ages of 8 and 20, it is then referred to as a nonossifying fibroma and must be differentiated from a unicameral bone cyst (23).

Case 5.8

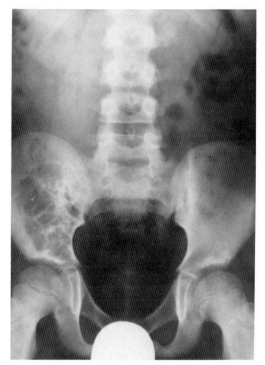

Fig. 5.8 A.   Kevin S.

Kevin is an 11-year-old "Rocket" football player. Last Saturday during a game he was blocked from behind, and later that evening he complained of low back discomfort.

On Monday he was brought in by his mother for examination. Moderate muscular spasm and tenderness was found at the L-S level bilaterally. Neurological and orthopedic testing were unrevealing. X-rays were done to rule out any possible fracture.

The final diagnosis of Kevin's injury was acute posttraumatic lumbosacral myofascial strain. Spinal manipulation, soft-tissue massage, initial cryotherapy followed by alternating moist heat packs, bed rest, and exercise brought prompt, uncomplicated relief.

Incidentally noted on Fig. 5.8, *A* and *B*, is a rather large bony lesion. What is it, and what should you do for it?

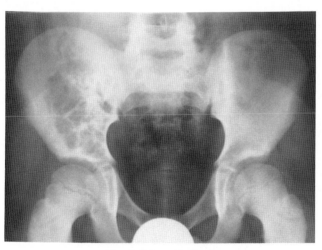

Fig. 5.8 B.   Kevin S.

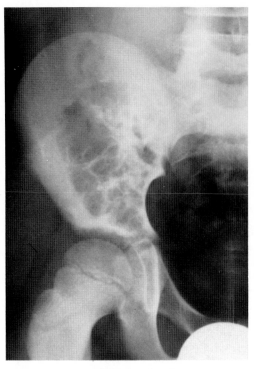

Fig. 5.8 C. Kevin S.

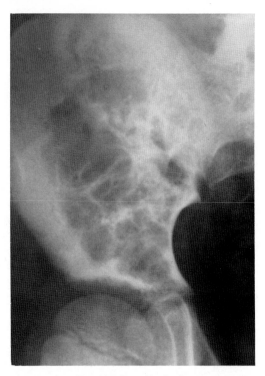

Fig. 5.8 D. Kevin S.

On the initial review a rather large accumulation of gas pattern was suspect over the left ilium. Careful inspection finds this pattern totally confined within the bone and not having typical colonic markings—definitely not gas.

The rather large area of radiolucency demonstrates with reasonably well defined margination and marked septal formation of accentuated trabeculation—a multiloculated appearance.

It is monostotic, i.e., involves only one bony site. While *fibrous dysplasia* often causes cortical thinning and expansion of bone, this typically is found in long bones. When seen in the flat bones, such as in the skull or ilium, the lesion tends towards a large cyst-like radiolucency with dense sclerotic margination or the heavy, thickened trabeculated or septal formation, as

seen in this case (13).

Fibrous dysplasia represents a developmental disturbance caused by a germ plasm defect producing abnormal proliferation of fibrous tissue. Variation in the degree and amount of bone contained within the lesion produces the radiographic alterations ranging from large cyst-like areas, to septal formations, to the "milky" or "ground glass" appearance seen usually in the extremities and in polystotic involvement. It is generally found incidentally, as in this case, and is of clinical concern due to its thinned cortex which may predispose towards pathological fracture. Limitation of activity or possible surgical intervention may be necessary, dependent on the size and site of involvement. The lesions tend to stabilize with adulthood (23).

Case 5.9

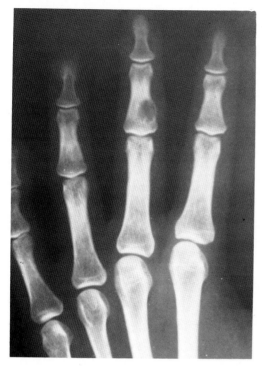

Fig. 5.9 A. Lamar J.

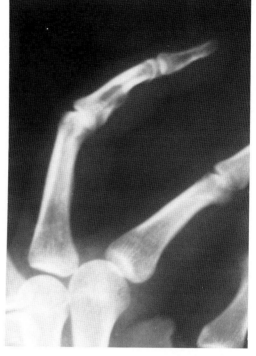

Fig. 5.9 B. Lamar J.

Lamar is a 32-year-old man who has been undergoing treatment for an unrelated illness. Quite casually he mentions that the middle finger of his left hand has become very sensitive to the touch with fleeting periods of slight pain. No significant soft-tissue swelling is noted, and no loss of sensory or motor function of the digit is reported.

On palpation, a hard, small, tender nodular area is noted of the proximal end of the third middle phalanx. It is nonmova-

ble. Joint function is not disturbed, although forced extension aggravates pain. Further examination and historical exploration are unrevealing.

Fig. 5.9, *A* and *B*, indicates the presence of the most common bone tumor of the hand. Do you remember what it is? What other similar lesions must be considered in your differential diagnosis? What is a common complication of this condition? What treatment do you recommend?

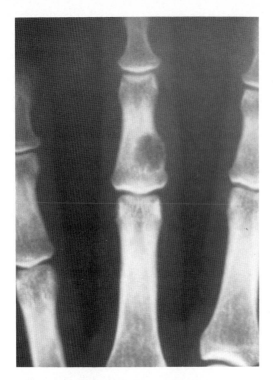

Fig. 5.9 C.   Lamar J.

The slow-growing solitary *enchondroma* is the most common benign bone tumor of the hand (13). Originating as a displaced cartilage rest, it is most often located within the medullary cavity of a bone. While occurring predominately as a single lesion, it is not infrequently found at multiple sites. The most favored sites are those of the distal aspects of the metacarpals and the proximal aspect of the phalanges, as in Lamar's case. Any bone preformed in cartilage may be involved. The lesion presents typically as a small round or ovoid lesion in short bones or, occasionally, with extensive involvement in the shaft of long bones.

The lesion may be seen as a well-demonstrated radiolucency which demonstrates with expansion. It does not cause cortical breakthrough except with pathological fracture, and does not evoke local periosteitis. Occasionally the lesion is well marginated with dense sclerotic thickening and may contain stippled or spotty calcific densities within.

An epidermoid inclusion cyst of a distal phalanx may present a differential challenge with the enchondroma. Expansile cortical breakthrough, a lack of calcific flecking, and a history of a penetrating trauma are characteristic of the inclusion cyst and often will aid in this differentiation (13).

Due to the attending loss of architectural integrity of the enchondroma, pathological fracture is frequent. Indeed it is often the initial reason for patient presentation for examination. The treatment most frequently employed is surgical curettage, followed by packing with bone chips.

Case 5.10

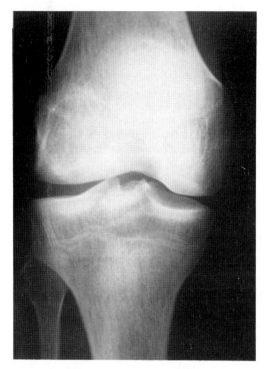

Fig. 5.10 A.   Peter N.

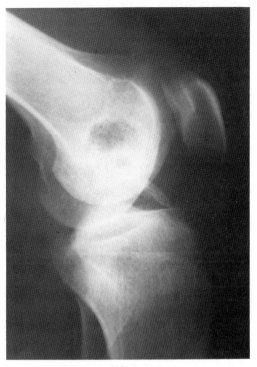

Fig. 5.10 B.   Peter N.

Peter is 20-year-old man who reports progressively worsening pain in his right knee. While an occasinal tennis player, he is really not athletically inclined. There is no history of severe or repetitive injury.

Slight swelling, weakness and moderate pain for the past two months is reported. Joint function has been only minimally disturbed. Joint "noise" of clicking is reported. Laboratory tests are normal, and neurological examination is unrevealing.

Fig. 5.10, *A*, *B* and *C*, indicates a well-defined, radiolucent, somewhat circular lesion which is eccentrically located at the distal end of the femur, near its margin. Noted on the lateral projection (Fig. 5.10*B*) is a dense streaking of chondrocalcinosis located near the anterior portion of the joint. No evidence of reactive periosteitis or destruction of contiguous bone is seen.

There are two likely diagnostic considerations of this lesion. Both are uncommon but are often discussed. Remember the lesion's location and make a stab at it!

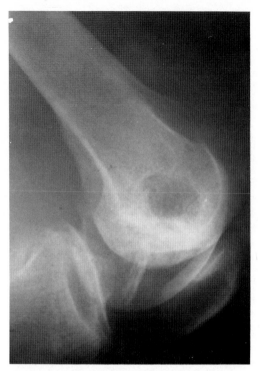

Fig. 5.10 C.   Peter N.

There are two tumors which are frequently located in the epiphysis of the distal femur and proximal tibia. In both the lesion is demonstrated off the central axis, i.e., eccentric, and tends to extend towards the articular plate.

While the giant cell tumor is considered as a quasimalignant tumor and is uncommon, the benign chondroblastoma is rather rare.

The giant cell tumor typically occurs in an older age group (20 to 40), is larger in size, has greater radiolucency and lacks the sharp margination and matrix calcification frequently noted in chondroblastoma (13).

The *benign chondroblastoma* in Peter's case is characterized by its epiphyseal location with slight metaphyseal extension. Its size is typical, although a smaller lesion is not uncommon. The round or oval radiolucency, with a thin sharply demarcated sclerotic margin eccentrically placed, is common for this neoplasm. Frequently, amorphous spotty calcifications are seen within the lesion, which help to identify its cartilaginous origin.

Clinically, as in Peter's case, pain is the predominant symptom and is referred to the involved joint. Benign chondroblastoma typically occurs in the 10 to 20 age group.

The joint clicking described by the patient was due to the chondrocalcinosis which is not typical of chondroblastoma but, because of its cartilaginous origin, not surprising. Direct extension from the tumor is doubtful.

Although some have suggested that benign chondroblastoma is a slow-growing malignant tumor, this is still debated (2). Treatment therefore continues to be generally of the more conservative approach via curettage with close observation for recurrence.

Case 5.11

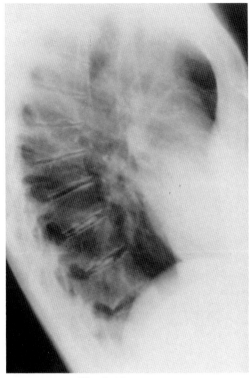

Fig. 5.11. Ann P.

Ann P. is a 32-year-old woman who presented with chronic generalized backache. No acute symptoms were recalled.

Ann reported that all her life people had been telling her to "stand up straight" but that nonetheless she had developed slouching posture. She apparently had attributed all back discomfort to posture and had never been radiographed until these films had been taken. No significant trauma was reported.

Clinically, a marked lumbar hyperlordosis and a moderate increase of the thoracic kyphosis were seen. No point tenderness or palpable muscular tension of significance was noted. There were no positive orthopedic or neurologic findings. Darkened urine was noted, particularly after standing.

Calcification of the intervertebral discs can be seen in Fig. 5.11. This is, in itself, not a sufficient diagnosis unless you have ruled out the few conditions which can produce/precipitate this cartilaginous calcification. What are they? We'll give you a hint, the patient's age is of significance.

Case 5.12

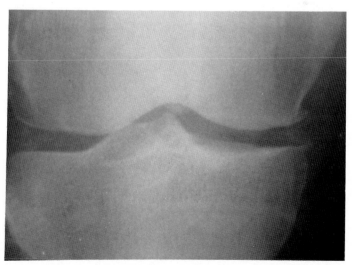

Fig. 5.12. Norma K.

In Fig. 5.12, notice the fine calcific streaking of the articular cartilage streaking of the articular cartilage and menisci.

This also represents cartilaginous calcification but of a different origin than that in Fig. 5.11.

The various articular cartilaginous calcifications (chondrocalcinosis) which are frequently encountered are the result of gout, hyperparathyroidism, pseudogout, degeneration and ochronosis.

To the above, those which affect the intervertebral disc as well include idiopathic, posttraumatic, ankylosing spondylitis and hypervitaminosis D.

Fig. 5.11 shows *ochronosis*. This condition is the result of altered metabolism of homogentisic acid, an inborn error. Due to this metabolic defect, deposition of oxydized homogentisic acid occurs in cartilage, causing pigmentation, degeneration and calcification. A propensity towards the intervertebral disc(s) is seen, although peripheral joints may also be involved due to abnormal accumulation of homogentisic acid in blood and urine. These high concentrations can produce very dark urine on voiding, which becomes black after standing or after it is alkalinized. While calcification of the intervertebral discs can occur with a simple degenerative process, this typically occurs in the older patient (22). In ochronosis, the patient is usually a young adult (25 to 35 years) and more frequently female. The condition does produce early degenerative discal thinning and typically eventuates into an early discogenic spondylosis. Calcification of the intervertebral discs, particularly if multiple involvement is seen in young adult female, should arouse the suspicion of ochronosis. Clinically, an increased thoracic kyphosis is frequently seen.

Fig. 5.12 demonstrates the fine calcific streaking within the articular cartilage and menisci quite typical of the chondrocalcinosis of the *pseudogout syndrome*. In this condition the deposition of calcium pyrophosphate crystals in articular joints and bursa is common, leading to calcification(s). While the symptoms are similar to gout, the serum uric acid levels are not elevated. The knee and wrist are the sites of preference in pseudogout, although a vertical streak of chondrocalcinosis within the symphysis pubis articulation is also frequently seen (13) (Fig. 5.13).

Case 5.13

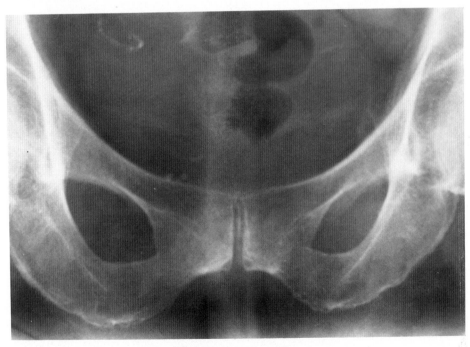

Fig. 5.13.   Myrna O.

Fig 5.13 shows vertical chondrocalcinosis within the pubic articulation. While possibly of pseudogout origin, the small cystic subchondral radiolucencies suggest probable degenerative origin.

Case 5.14

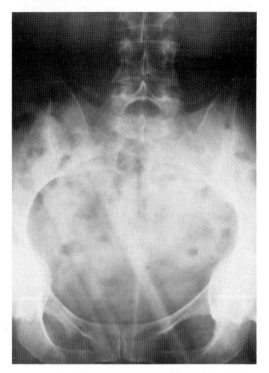

Fig. 5.14 A. Caroline M.

Caroline is a 42-year-old woman who has born one child, 12 years ago. Although the pregnancy was uneventful, she had been prepared to face a possible dystocia or painful delivery. Preparation was made for cesarean section delivery, but fortunately all went well and a normal delivery was achieved.

Over the past few years she has noted progressive difficulty with hip mobility—mostly stiffness. Lately her family has noticed that she has begun to limp. Some dull ache has been noted with stress or fatigue.

Last week Caroline noticed that the pain developed in her hips and low back after crossing one knee over the other. Both sides seemed equally affected. The discomfort was localized and disappeared when she resumed normal posture. No edema, paresthesias or atrophy have been noted.

All orthopedic tests were bilaterally positive for hip joint involvement. Neurological examination, however, was noncontributory. Radiography was done, and after review, laboratory tests were considered unnecessary at this time.

Caroline has enjoyed generally good health. She denies any psoriasis or skin disorders. There is no familial history of tuberculosis. She has always been quite active, having been a cheerleader in both high school and college, and has never been physically limited or restricted.

The condition which Caroline has is relatively rare but occurs frequently enough and is sufficiently interesting to be included for your enjoyment. (A learning experience is, after all, fun, isn't it?) Is this condition developmental, traumatic or pathological?

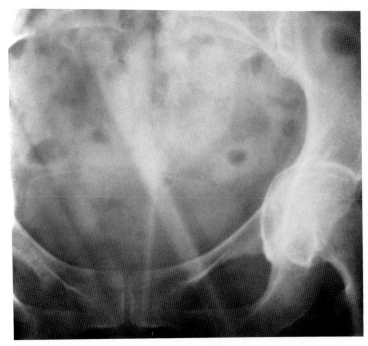

Fig. 5.14 *B*.   Caroline M.

The condition which Caroline has is referred to as arthrokatadysis, protrusio acetabuli or, most commonly, *Otto pelvis*. Described originally by Otto and Krobak, it refers to the bilateral protrusion of the femoral head and acetabulum into the pelvis. The developmental form occurs during childhood and adolescence and often remains undetected (19).

A traumatic form is suggested due to interference of development on a nutritional basis. A purely traumatic form is possible with rupture of the femoral head(s) through the acetabula in the adult. A pathological basis is found in any case of severely destructive arthritis which erodes the roof of the acetabulum, i.e., psoriatic, rheumatoid or tubercular arthritis, or in those disease processes which allow for the weight-bearing thrust of the femoral head to break through the acetabula, i.e., Paget's disease or severe osteomalacia (22).

It is recognized that in most of the unilateral or pathological protrusions, the correct term of intrapelvic protrusion of the acetabulum is preferred—the Otto pelvis remaining descriptive of a developmental bilateral protrusion.

With progression of the aging process, the Otto pelvis predisposes to early degenerative joint disease. Mobility becomes limited particularly in abduction and external rotation. A hip flexion deformity may occur, causing secondary pelvic rotation and increased lumbar lordosis. Thereafter, biomechanical dysfunction of the lumbopelvic complex is frequently encountered.

Our concern with Caroline's pregnancy relates to the frequent dystocia which occurs when this condition is severe enough to cause encroachment of the pelvic birth canal. The Otto pelvis occurs mainly in women.

Case 5.15

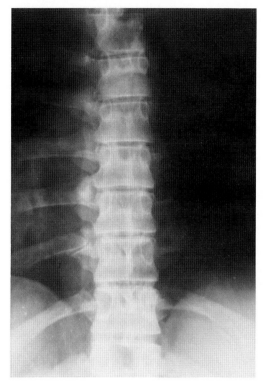

Fig. 5.15 A. David H.

David H. reported having had pain in the midthoracic spine for the previous two years. The pain was constant, although worse at night, sharpened with certain postural stresses, and had been unyielding to many varied medications. His only relief, and the only way he was comfortable enough to sleep, was by using aspirin.

Coughing and sneezing tended to aggravate the pain, and he had allergic responses to ragweed. This combination made the patient extremely apprehensive for fear of pain aggravation.

Interestingly, numerous radiographs had been taken at various facilities without an adequate diagnosis being determined.

Clinically, all orthopedic and neurological testing was essentially unremarkable. Some moderate paraspinal tension was noted on palpation to the left of midline from T6 through T10. The patient was mesomorphic in appearance, somewhat apprehensive, and reported a weight loss of ten pounds over the preceding six months. He was, needless to say, quite frustrated over the lack of appropriate diagnosis and treatment.

With careful review of a good quality radiograph (Fig. 5.15A), this case presents the classic appearance of the condition affecting David. You of course have the diagnosis well in hand by now, right? What is your recommended treatment?

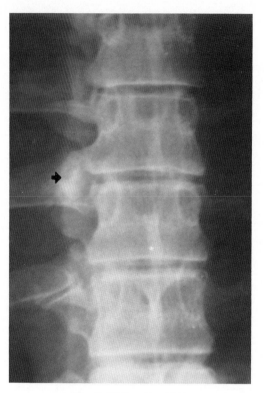

Fig. 5.15 *B*.   David H.

A dense, radiopaque ovoid structure is noted within the proximal head of the eighth posterior rib on the left (see *arrow* on Fig. 5.15B). By its size and location it is definitely not a part of the vertebra or transverse process.

The well-defined margins of the lesion suggest benignity, and careful inspection reveals a radiolucent centrum within.

This radiolucent nidus, surrounded by a dense, reactive, sclerotic well-marginated lesion is typical of an *osteoid osteoma* (13).

While the nidus is often obscured by the sclerotic reaction all around it, in this case it is nicely identifiable.

When only a dense sclerotic lesion is seen, the need for tomographic examination is in order to demonstrate the nidus for diagnostic confirmation.

The osteoid osteoma is a common lesion found twice as often in males than in females and usually in patients under 25. The most common site of involvement is the femur and tibia, but it is frequently seen in the fibula, humerus, vertebral arch, and spinous and transverse processes. Now that we've said that, it's time to tell you also that David is 42 and that his osteoid osteoma was located in the proximal rib head. So much for statistics!

The typical treatment for this condition is surgical curettement and packing with bone chips. In this case, already unusual by site and age of occurrence, the surgical team found a rather extensive cartilaginous extension or root which was directed anteriorly and downward towards the posterior cardiac wall. The lesion was curetted and packed with most of the extension removed, but the distal end was left in place in fear of creating pericardial rection. Although a slower-than-typical response was encountered, the patient did in time have abatement of symptoms.

Case 5.16

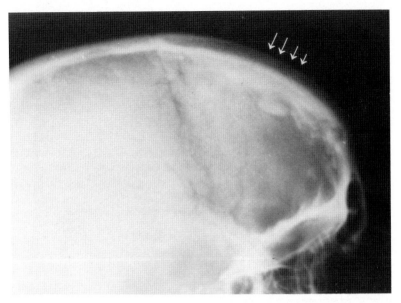

Fig. 5.16A. Ava C.

Ava is a 54-year-old Caucasian woman who suffers from recurrent headaches, the result of intermittent vasospasm of the vertebral artery and moderately severe covertebral joints of Luschka arthrosis. Fig. 5.16A was taken following an acute sinusitis. The findings are therefore incidental. Notice the thickened, sclerotic appearance of the frontal region. The outer table (*arrows*) has not been broken or significantly expanded. The frontal sinus is clear.

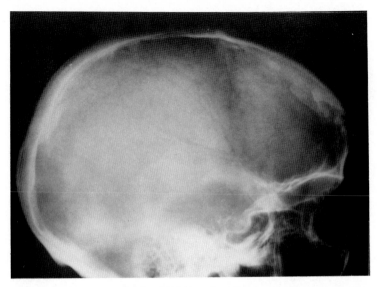

Fig. 5.16 *B*. Ava C.

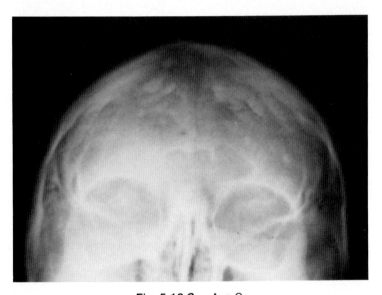

Fig. 5.16 *C*. Ava C.

The area of patchy, dense sclerotic bony proliferation shown in Fig. 5.16A is characteristic of hyperostosis. It is confined to the frontal bone and to the internal table of the skull. The diploë are not affected. Known as *hyperostosis frontalis interna*, it is a peculiar overgrowth of bone found principally in the postmenopausal woman (20). The condition is one of disputed clinical importance but has been implicated as a possible sign of endocrine imbalance.

One of the more important differential signs, aside from those described above, is that the hyperostosis surrounds the venous sinuses but does not obliterate them (23).

B and *C* of Fig. 5.16 are of the same patient one year later. No significant change in the amount or degree of hyperostosis is seen.

The condition is totally asymptomatic and does not induce alterations of routine laboratory findings.

Case 5.17

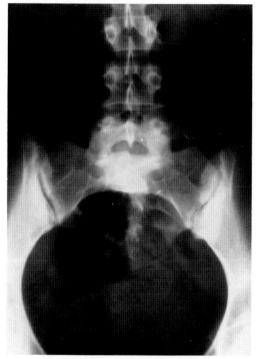

Fig. 5.17 A.   Annie D.

Annie is a 24-year-old woman who reports a constant, dull ache of her low back. No significant history of trauma is reported. No painful radiations or paresthesis into the lower extremities have occurred.

The discomfort usually follows prolonged sitting or standing and is relieved with bed rest.

Annie is a housewife and mother, with four children ranging in age from six weeks to six years. She reports that the present complaint appeared gradually over the past three or four months. While denying prior low back problems, she does remember a similar discomfort a couple of years ago, soon after the birth of her third child. At that time, no treatment was sought, and abatement of symptoms was spontaneous within a few weeks.

Examination indicates palpable tenderness with moderate muscular rigidity of the lumbosacral and sacroiliac areas, more so on the right. No other positive orthopedic, neurological or laboratory findings have been uncovered.

From the above history and Fig. 5.17A, you should be able to identify this somewhat innocuous, benign condition. What is the anticipated course of treatment, and will sequelae develop?

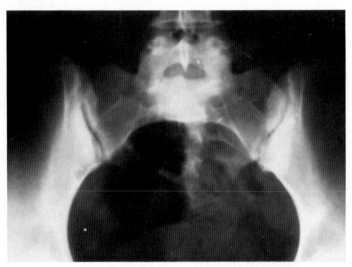

Fig. 5.17 B.   Annie D.

A zone of dense sclerosis is noted in Fig. 5.17, *A* and *B*, along the iliac side of the sacroiliac articulations, bilaterally. The interarticular joint space is well maintained, and the sacrum has escaped involvement. The condition is termed *osteitis condensans ilii*; its etiology is unclear. Found frequently in pregnancy or in postparturition, it appears related to the abnormal stresses and strains to the sacroiliac joints during pregnancy and delivery. The clinical picture of Annie is typical, and many cases of osteitis condensans ilii are found incidentally in the search for other problems. The lesions probably abate spontaneously and rarely provide sequelae of importance (22). The zone of sclerosis is presumably due to abnormal stress, and once the stress is removed, return to normal architecture is anticipated. The condition is usually bilateral and symmetrical, although variation in intensity between the two sides does occur.

Occasionally this condition must be differentiated from rheumatoid arthritis and ankylosing spondylitis. These latter conditions affect the joint space and articular surface of the bones on both sides of the joint. Typically, the joint margins become blurred and eventually become ankylosed. Ankylosing spondylitis affects young males predominately, with a male/female ratio of approximately 15:1.

The small, beaded semicircular radiopacity located just inferior to the zone of condensation on the left is a screen artifact.

Case 5.18

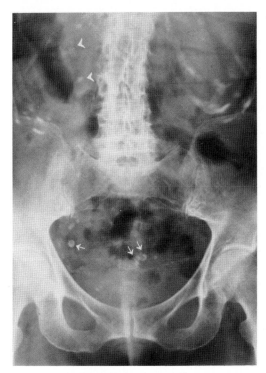

Fig. 5.18A. Jane D.

Jane's clinical problem relates to postural and emotional stresses which are not an issue radiographically. Her films are presented due to several interesting findings which you might find helpful.

The patient is a 43-year-old woman, an elementary school teacher who denies any history of prior injury or serious illness. She has always been thin, athletically inclined and maintains good muscular tone. She has never been pregnant. No history of kidney infection or stones and only occasional dysmenorrhea are reported. All laboratory tests are normal.

You will note that at the two *arrowheads* in Fig. 5.18A, several somewhat circular radiopacities are barely discernible. Due to their size and location the possibility of renal calculi must be considered. Fortunately for Jane the lateral film (Fig. 5.18B) demonstrates these areas to be located in the anterior sector, and therefore the kidney examination is not necessary. The remaining calcifications are the areas in question.

The *arrows* located in the true pelvis point to circular radiopacities of varying size. These scattered, well-defined radiodensities are typical of *calcified phleboliths*. These are frequently encountered, mostly in females, and are thought to relate to prior pelvic inflammation or infection. They represent calcification of a small venous thrombus with the calcium deposits in the wall of the vein. When seen, they are of little clinical importance. Historically they may shed light on some prior pelvic disorder overlooked by the patient.

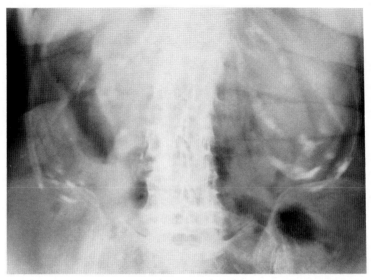

Fig. 5.18 B. Jane D. If Jane had been 63 instead of 43, this film would have probably been overlooked.

Case 5.19

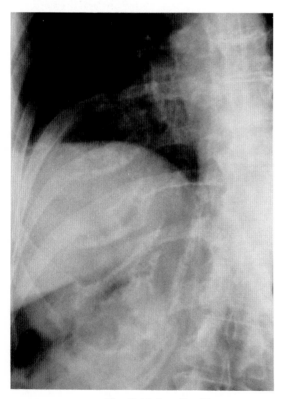

Fig. 5.18 C. Eva T.

This degree of *costochondral calcification* is frequently found in the aged.

Generally considered a normal finding, the calcification is characteristically mottled in appearance and can at times be quite extensive. It is well to remember that the costal cartilage is not normally seen on x-ray unless calcification has occurred.

Most of the literature we've read suggests that this condition is the result of general aging or previous trauma. One thing seems certain—only a select few seem to develop this condition, regardless of etiology. It is progressive as a rule, at times involving all of the costal cartilages. With calcification comes loss of rib excursion. This loss may be of clinical concern in cases of limited respiratory function and in severe scoliotics (21).

It is problematical if costochondral calcification should be considered more than an incidental finding. With its propensity towards development in the aged and, at least in our own experience, its being found more frequently in the female than in the male, we cannot help but ponder a possible hormonal relationship.

In Fig. 5.18C is seen the typical appearance of costochondral calcification. Eva is a 62-year-old woman. Notice the flocculent, mottled appearance as the calcifications silhouette the anterior costochondral structures.

Case 5.20

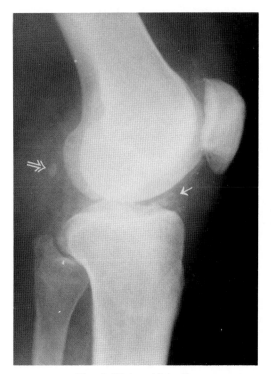

Fig. 5.19 A. Mary P.

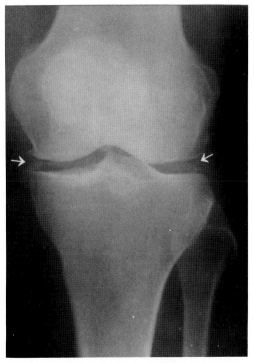

Fig. 5.19 B. Mary P.

Mary is a 61-year-old Caucasian woman who reports frequent episodes of pain and swelling of her right knee. The symptoms tend to occur spontaneously and dissipate on their own every three or four months. The duration of acute pain is usually six to ten days. She has never had similar complaints involving her feet. The current findings include pain, tenderness, slight swelling and suggested joint heat. Labora-tory findings include normal levels of se-rum calcium, phosphorus, alkaline phos-phatase, uric acid and homogentisic acid.

The *single arrows* on Fig. 5.19, *A* and *B*, are directed to what characteristic feature of Mary's condition? What is the *double arrow* directed towards? Is there another name for this condition when asympto-matic?

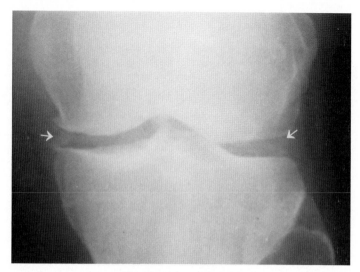

Fig. 5.19 C. Mary P.

The *single arrows* in Fig. 5.19 of Mary's knee are directed to the fine calcific streaking of the menisci and articular cartilage. This finding when coupled with the clinical symptoms described, yet lacking an elevated serum uric acid level, is characteristic of *pseudogout*. In contrast to gout in which uric acid crystals are deposited in articular cartilage, pseudogout refers to the deposition of calcium pyrophosphate crystals in joints and bursae. The clinical symptoms are similar. The knee and wrist are most frequently involved as opposed to the metatarsophalangeal joint, a favored site in gout (11, 12, 18).

Definitive demonstration of the calcium pyrophosphate crystals may be done via needle biopsy, but extrapolative differentiation is sufficient by clinical and laboratory findings as described.

When asymptomatic, this radiographic finding is referred to as chondrocalcinosis—that's what you called it in the first place, right?

The *double arrow* in Fig. 5.19A is directed towards the fabella, a normal sesamoid bone.

Case 5.21

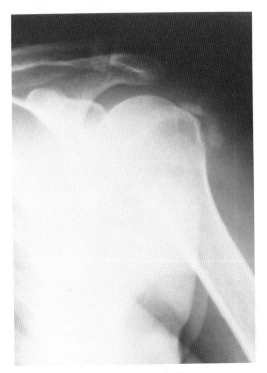

Fig. 5.20. Doris S.

Doris, a 38-year-old Caucasian woman, developed severe pain in her right shoulder about three days ago. She reports that the shoulder has bothered her periodically for three to four months.

Clinically, there was no fever, no history of gout, no significant erythema and little soft-tissue edema. She was unable to abduct the arm without producing great pain, i.e., painful arc of movement. Palpable point tenderness was noted over the greater tubercle and overlying deltoid muscle.

Various authors have called the condition shown in Fig. 5.20 by numerous terms; are you familiar with the correct one? A

variety of this condition, when affecting the medial collateral ligament of the knee, is referred to as Pellegrini-Stieda disease. The condition is frequently associated with overuse or trauma of the involved joint.

In Doris S.'s case (Fig. 5.20), had you referred to this as calcified subdeltoid bursitis, calcific rotator cuff tendinitis or calcific tendinitis of the supraspinatus, you would find much agreement and disagreement. The exact pathogenesis of this condition is not fully understood. Assumption is made that trauma or degenerative change produces small tears or ruptures in the ligamentous and tendinous fibrils with associated hemorrhages, necrosis and subsequent deposits of calcium. The calcific deposits are initially in the tendon and work their way towards the surface, rupturing the floor of the bursa. Prior to its bursting into the bursa, the calcific deposit produces acute irritation to the bursa, i.e., acute bursitis. Should thickening of the bursa as the result of adhesion formation occur, a chronic bursitis is found. Once the calcific material enters into the bursa, it is absorbed and spontaneous remission of symptoms occurs. Recurrent attacks of calcific deposits with irritation of the overlying bursa may result in a chronic adhesive bursitis (22).

Because the radiograph is rarely definitive as to the exact location of the calcific deposit, i.e., pericapsular tendons, ligaments or bursae, the all-inclusive term *peritendinitis calcarea* has been adopted. It is often necessary to secure radiographs with rotated views of the humerus to define the calcific deposits adequately. Some suggest a lessened kilovolts peak technique. The demonstration of osteoporosis of the greater tubercle is considered a localized sign of chronicity.

Case 5.22

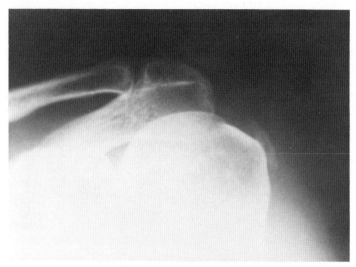

Fig. 5.21. Myrtle B.

Myrtle B.'s case (Fig. 5.21) is another example of *peritendinitis calcarea.* The amount of calcific deposit in Myrtle's case is less than that in Doris S.'s case, but the degree of clinical pain and discomfort is the same. This condition developed suddenly but was thought to be related to occupational stress of repetitive pulling on a manual stamping press at work.

Case 5.23

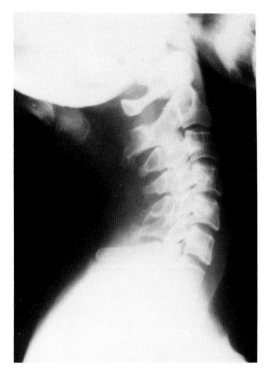

Fig. 5.22 A. Linda L.

Linda, a 19-year-old woman, is a member of an olympic volleyball team. For a serious player like Linda, the intensity of the sport is much different from what is usually associated with volleyball as played at picnics and family outings. During practice recently she was hit with the ball several times about the base of her head and neck. The next day, much stiffness with some soft-tissue swelling was noted. Examination revealed a moderate myofascial cervical strain but of concern was the palpatory findings of two hardened masses located at the skull base just left of midline.

After review of Fig. 5.22, *A, B* and *C,* Linda was questioned further. She recalled being knocked unconscious eight weeks previously when, during match play, another player accidentally hit the base of her head—instead of the ball! (What a passing shot that would have been!) That night, much soft-tissue swelling was noted. Contusion and bruising were present for about one week and then eventually dissipated, although residual tension was noted when combing her hair. The recent hit aggravated the tenderness.

You will note that the cervical spine itself is normal. Range of motion is limited in hyperextension (above) due to soft-tissue insult. Two rather large radiopaque structures are noted near the external occipital protuberance. What type of density is noted, and does it have any characteristic form? Can you remember the diagnostic term which is appropriate?

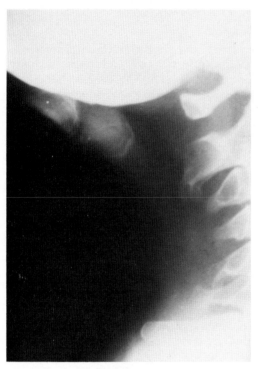

Fig. 5.22 B.   Linda L.

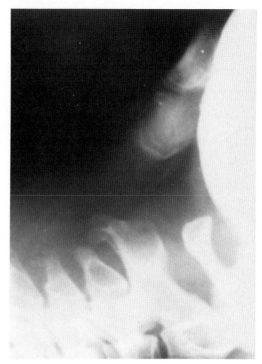

Fig. 5.22 C.   Linda L.

Following severe soft-tissue trauma to the deep tissues, a hematoma often results. This is frequent in athletes but may be encountered in any local injury severe enough to cause deep tissue bruising of the muscle with or without frank hemorrhage. Calcification of the hematoma follows. Initially it is seen radiographically as a dense hazy shadow of increased density. Over a period of several weeks this becomes denser and eventually develops the appearance of bone.

The lesion typically has a laminated appearance caused by the hemorrhage dissecting along the muscle planes. Usually after a prolonged period of time, resorption occurs, and the ossification gradually decreases in size. Smaller masses may disappear completely. Occasionally the original injury is severe enough to also produce similar findings in the periosteum imme-

diately beneath the injured area. Rarely, osteogenic sarcoma has developed. The condition is most frequently seen in the thigh muscles of football players. It is referred to as *posttraumatic myositis ossificans*.

The heterotopic soft-tissue calcification of myositis ossificans has three distinct etiologies. Progressive myositis ossificans is a genetic dysplasia in which congenital osseous abnormalities are associated with progressive soft-tissue ossification. It begins in the very young, is not associated with trauma, and progresses until the entire body becomes fixed and immobile. In myositis ossificans associated with neurological diseases, extensive soft-tissue ossifications are present, particularly in the para-articular regions, leading to ankylosis of the joints. The condition develops below the level of the neurological lesion (12, 23).

Case 5.24

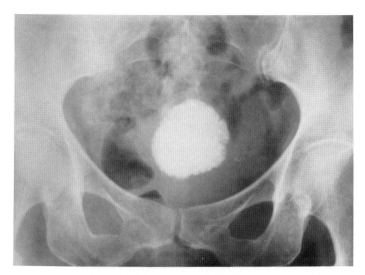

Fig. 5.23. Marie M.

Marie is a 68-year-old Caucasian woman who injured her low back in a fall.

The lesion shown in Fig. 5.23 was found incidental to examination. Note the rather large, homogeneous circular radiopacity located at midpelvis. While the lesion is well defined, the margin presents with a "mulberry type" appearance.

Is this lesion benign or malignant, and what does it represent?

Case 5.25

Alice, a 57-year-old black woman, also presented with an interesting incidental finding.

The lesion shown in Fig. 5.24 is heterogeneous, located just right of midline, and has a somewhat irregular margin. Its overall density, however, is of calcific radiopacity. The "mulberry type" appearance is more pronounced in this case.

Answer the same questions about Alice's case that were asked about in Marie's case.

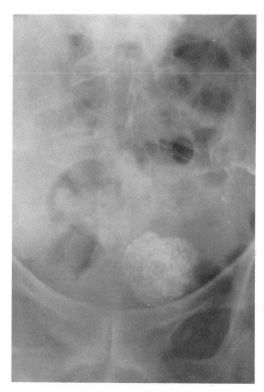

Fig. 5.24. Alice G.

The well-defined calcific lesion shown in Fig. 5.23 represents a *calcified uterine fibroma*. The dense radiopacity is characteristic, as is the central or midpelvis location. The well-defined margination indicates benignity. While it is a space-occupying lesion, the calcified uterine fibroma is rarely of clinical importance and seldom, if ever, undergoes malignant degeneration. Occasionally, should the lesion occupy the entire pelvis, compression of surrounding structures may require surgical removal.

Alice G.'s case is another example *calcified uterine fibroma*. Fig. 5.24 demonstrates much less calcification, but the size, location and "mulberry type" appearance of the fibroma are typical (23). While

somewhat irregular, the margin remains intact, indicating benignity. The heterogeneous appearance is due to a more "spotty" deposition of calcium.

In both of these cases, uterine fibromas which have undergone calcification as the result of tumoral metaplasia are seen. This same process can and does occur in *ovarian fibroids* (see Fig. 5.25). These calcified tumors are characteristically smaller and farther from the midpelvis, i.e., lateral due to anatomical size and location. It is frequently difficult to differentiate the two on plain film radiographs, but the history of uterine versus ovarian disease is helpful. Both types are generally not of clinical importance when achieving this degree of calcification.

Case 5.26

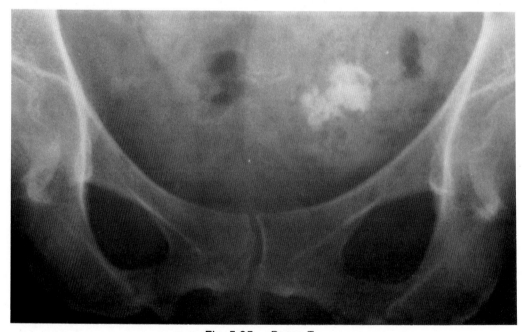

Fig. 5.25.   Peggy T.

Peggy is a 60-year-old woman who relates a long history of menstrual problems, including dysmenorrhea and repetitive infection for many years prior to menopause.

The *calcified ovarian fibroma* is well demonstrated in the right midpelvis and is characteristically less well marginated than the uterine fibromata.

Case 5.27

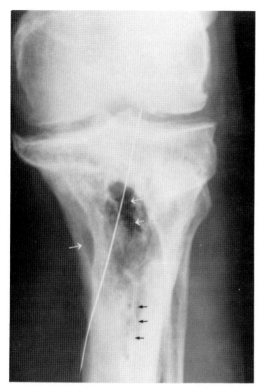

Fig. 5.26 A. Otto B.

Otto, a World War I veteran, has a draining lesion of the anteromedial aspect of the tibia. Marked brownish induration involves the upper one third of the leg. The drainage site has opened and closed spontaneously for years.

History reveals that originally Otto had been hit with shrapnel and treated with sulfur powder. The wound has never healed. He has been advised many times in subsequent years to undergo amputation, but has refused. The last 50 years or so have been a continuous battle of periodic medication, dressings, discomfort and limited activities. He has been able to work as an accountant, however, without great distress.

When he presented for examination and treatment, the lesion was obvious. Diminished reflexes, some moderate muscular atrophy, and coldness of the lower leg and foot were found. No fever, edema, intermittent claudication or paresthesias were demonstrated. Laboratory work indicated *slight* elevation in ESR, alkaline phosphatase and WBC count. Minimal normochromic, normocytic anemia was found. The patient was lethargic. The specific etiological agent has never been adequately established, but either staphylococcus or streptococcal organisms seem logical.

Several classical findings typically associated with this chronic condition are seen in Fig. 5.26A (*arrows*). Can you identify each and remember their significance? This condition is somewhat rare today. Why?

In case you wondered about the long, slender, *vertical white line* on Fig. 5.26A, it's an artifact.

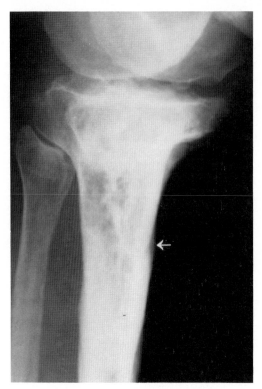

Fig. 5.26 B. Otto B.

Otto suffers with *chronic osteomyelitis.* Fortunately this condition is not often seen today since the advent of appropriate medication. While the acute form is still very much a part of clinical practice, early and appropriate treatment usually prevents this chronic stage from developing.

The laboratory work, history and examination provide a picture of low-grade chronic infection. Otto's refusal to accept anything except short-term treatment explains the chronic clinical picture.

The *upper two white arrows* in Fig. 5.26A indicate an area of radiolucency, suggesting cavitation with little evidence of reactive sclerosis or margination. This area represents the site of septic necrosis which still contains pus along with bony debris. The *single white arrow* in Fig. 5.26, A and B, indicates a sinus or fistula tract formation known as cloaca, through which drainage of the lesion occurs to the outside. The cloaca penetrates the shell of new bone formed by the periosteum in an attempt to seal off the lesion. This new bone formation is termed the involucrum (12, 19).

The *black arrows* in Fig. 5.26A point out a few of the dense, chalky white areas of dead bone scattered throughout the lesion. These areas of dead bone or debris are known as the sequestrum. Because the pieces of dead bone are surrounded by granulation tissue, they stand out as chalky white.

You will also note the deformity of the proximal tibial metaphysis and the presence of degenerative joint disease of the knee with chondrocalcinosis.

Case 5.28

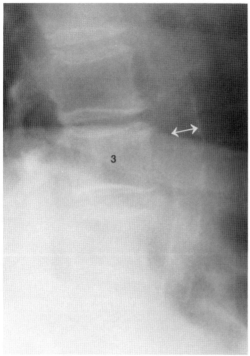

Fig. 5.27 A.   Janice P.

Janice P. is a 69-year-old Caucasian woman who reports with long-standing dull aching of the low back. She has had gradual loss of energy and tendency to be cold, particularly of the hands and feet.

Vital signs are a blood pressure of 174/88, a pulse pressure of 86, a pulse rate of 72, a temperature 98.8° and a respiratory rate of 16 to 18. She is 5 foot 4 inches tall and weights 146 pounds. Laboratory tests reveal slight cholesterolemia.

Your review of Fig. 5.27 A indicates moderate discogenic spondylosis of L2-L3. A tendency towards hyperextension subluxation of L3 on L4 is also noted. These findings would account for the recurrent back ache but would not adequately explain the suggested poor circulation and loss of energy.

The *white double-ended arrow* locates what structure? What process is ongoing, and does it explain the remaining clinical complaints? What other possible conditions would be suspect with this finding? Is it physiological or pathological?

Case 5.29

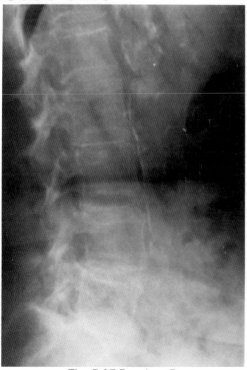

Fig. 5.27 B.   Amy D.

Amy is a 71-year-old widow who, despite her age, is quite active in civic affairs. She reports that just recently she has felt as though she were slowing down. She has become aware of a "throbbing" near her spine while lying down. Examination did not reveal any pulsating masses within the abdomen—a highly suggestive sign of aneurysm if found.

After review of Fig. 5.27, *A* and *B*, and the histories, which patient would you monitor most closely and why?

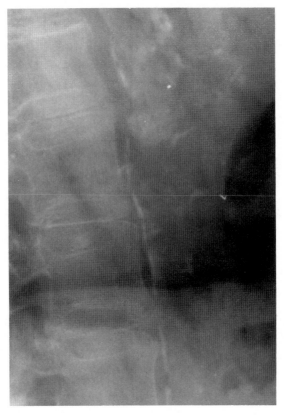

Fig. 5.27 C. Amy D.

Both Janice and Amy present with moderately extensive *atherosclerotic* plaqueing of the *abdominal aorta*. Considered a physiological process, from a clinical standpoint it is indeed pathophysiological. The elevated cholesterolemia is characteristic. (Be certain that all cholesterol determinations are taken after fasting.)

As the abdominal aorta is a rather large caliber vessel, it is probable that should the plaqueing process be noted here, other smaller vessels would also be involved. Indeed, this finding should suggest arteriosclerotic heart disease (AHD).

The combination of moderate elevation in blood pressure, overweight and cholesterolemia is highly suggestive of AHD. It would explain the fatigue and sluggish circulation.

With plaqueing comes a loss of tensile integrity and increased friability and fragility of the vessel. This predisposes to the production of arteriosclerotic aortic aneurysm. This, however, is not absolute; i.e., not every case of atherosclerotic abdominal aorta develops aneurysm, but it is frequent enough to warrant periodic monitoring. For determining an aneurysm, a fusiform dilatation should be noted. Neither patient presents with an aneurysm at this time. Remember too that the abdominal aorta bifurcates at the level of L4 into the right and left iliac arteries.

As noted in Fig. 5.27C, Amy's descending aorta is markedly tortuous with irregular plaqueing. The lack of marginal plaqueing on the anterior wall below the level of L2, in the presence of dilatation, suggests a possible thinning of the vessel wall. Coupled with the clinical symptoms, this indicates a need for close monitoring.

Case 5.30

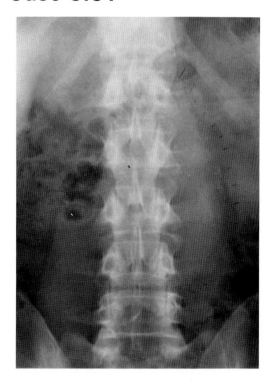

Fig. 5.28. Sheldon H.

Case 5.31

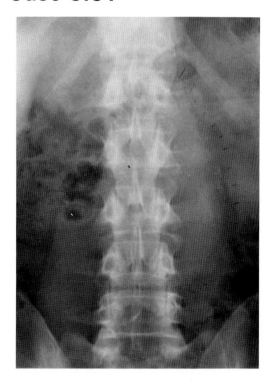

Fig. 5.29. Arthur C.

Sheldon, a 62-year-old colleague, had not felt well for some time. Reluctantly he sought consultation when a noticeable pulsation of his abdomen appeared, particularly when lying down.

Physical examination revealed a palpable, pulsating mass of the upper midabdomen. Radiographic examination was conclusive.

The lateral view seen in Fig. 5.28 reveals a large balloon-like fusiform swelling of the descending aorta, extending from the level of L2 through L4. The rather abrupt end of the distal portion indicates the point of aortic bifurcation.

The degree of calcification within the walls of this *abdominal aneurysm* indicates the slow progression and development of this lesion. In cases of rapid onset,

the walls are less well defined by plaqueing, and one must rely on variation of radiographic densities to define the size and shape of the aneurysm. While the size of the aneurysm may vary, when the A-P measurement exceeds 3.8 cm, dilatation is probable and should be regarded as significant. When the measurement exceeds 5.0 cm, the prognosis is grave (19).

On the AP radiograph an aneurysm of the distal aorta with calcification typically presents left of midline (see the radiograph of Arthur C., Fig. 5.29). This is often a helpful differential finding when other retroperitoneal lesions are being considered (19, 23).

Vigorous manipulation of the lumbar spine and pelvis is contraindicated in the presence of aneurysm of the distal aorta.

Case 5.32

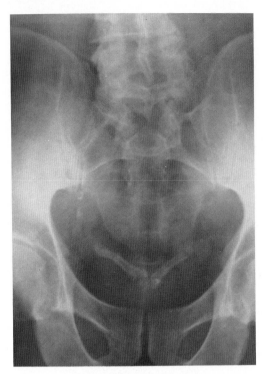

Fig. 5.30 A. Marty M.

Marty is a 56-year-old man whose clinical complaints are unrelated to this discussion. Historically, he has had a long-standing case of diabetes. No recorded prostatitis or chronic urinary bladder infections are reported.

Calcification of the vas deferens is occasionally seen in the older diabetic male. It rarely occurs in the nondiabetic. While being described as a degenerative phenomenon in these patients, its true etiology is unclear (23). The finding is more of a curiosity than a clinical concern, except to shed possible light on a long-standing history of diabetes.

Radiographically, the presence of densely calcified tubular shadows is seen. These shadows are generally bilateral and symmetrical, located in the lower midpelvis.

The directional angle, i.e., towards midline, helps to differentiate from atherosclerotic plaqueing of pelvic blood vessels of the same size, which tend towards lateral obliquity.

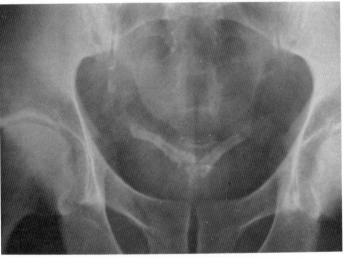

Fig. 5.30 B. Marty M.

Case 5.33

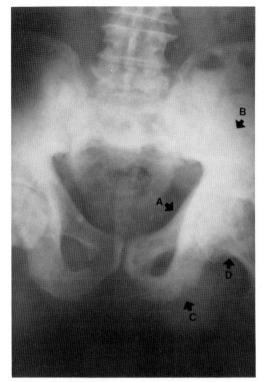

Fig. 5.31 A. Percy P.

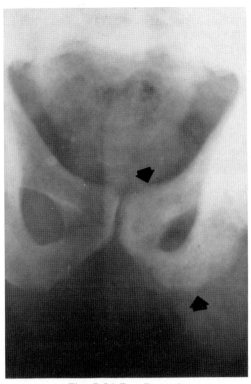

Fig. 5.31 B. Percy P.

Percy is a 57-year-old man who presented with dull headache and bone pain of the low back. Physical examination was inconclusive. These radiographs (Fig. 5.31, A and B) were obtained to help you arrive at your diagnosis, but certain laboratory tests are required for confirmation.

Before jumping to a conclusion, answer the following: Are the radiographs themselves of sufficient quality to allow adequate diagnosis? What x-ray findings do you see that are characteristic of the condition, and do these occur in any other condition? What laboratory findings would you order for your differential work-up?

Fig. 5.31A, an AP view of the pelvis, shows marked loss of bone detail and trabeculation on the right. The lumbar spine, however, demontrates excellent marginal detail. Because it is improbable to lose bony detail on only part of the film due to radiographic factors, we are assured that the film itself is OK. The variation must be in the bone itself.

At *arrow A* is seen a softened, thickened appearance of the pelvic brim. No reactive periosteitis is seen. At *arrow B*, loss of the trabecular pattern, with scattered areas of dense osteosclerosis, is seen throughout the right ilium. In Fig. 5.31B and at *arrow C* of Fig. 5.31A, loss of cortical definition is noted due to bony expansion of both the right ischial and pubic rami. Compare the size of the two, right and left. At *arrow D* in Fig. 5.31A, markedly thickened trabecular patterns, with accentuation of the criss-cross pattern, are seen within the femoral neck. This pattern is referred to as fasciculation and is also noted in Fig. 5.31C.

The rather dense, osteosclerotic pelvis with loss of trabecular and architectural detail is often seen in osteoblastic metastasis from the prostate. It also occurs in *Paget's disease*. The expansion of bone, softening of cortical margination, and fasciculation are characteristic of Paget's disase. Osteoblastic carcinoma from the prostate frequently involves the entire pelvis, while Paget's disease is often monostotic, as in this case.

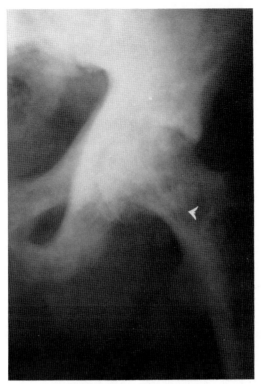

Fig. 5.31 C.   Percy P.

The laboratory findings are most helpful in the differentiation of metastatic prostatic carcinoma from Paget's disease. In prostatic metastasis an elevated serum *acid* phosphatase will be found, while in Paget's a markedly elevated serum *alkaline* phosphatase is usually encountered. In Paget's this can reach levels as high as 10 to 20 times normal. In those cases, estimated at 10 percent, where malignant degeneration from Paget's into osteosarcoma occurs, a dramatic rise in this already-elevated serum alkaline phosphatase will occur (2, 12).

The characteristics of this form of Paget's disease are summarized as cortical thickening with enlargement, softening of bone with dense osteosclerosis, and accentuation of the trabecular definition.

Case 5.34

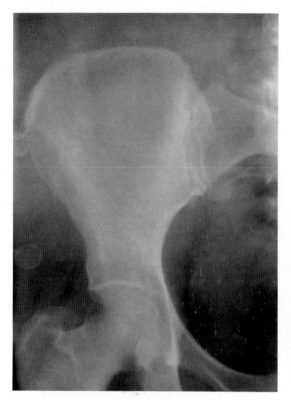

Fig. 5.32 A. Darlene D.

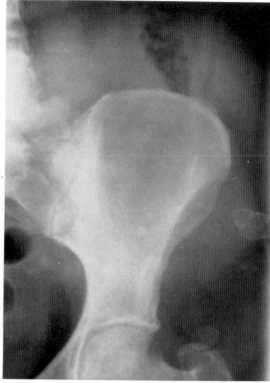

Fig. 5.32 B. Darlene D.

Case 5.34 is entered for its curiosity value and your general radiographic knowledge.

Darlene is a 36-year-old woman who, among a host of clinical problems, suffers with Addison's disease. Accordingly she has received numerous injections, primarily of cortisone, over the years. As a result the soft tissues of the buttock contain numerous somewhat circular *calcifications* *at the site of prior injection.* These radi- opacities are usually not as numerous as seen in Fig. 5.32, but you should be able to recognize them when seen. The calcifica- tions are of little clinical importance and must not be confused with other more significant soft-tissue calcifications. Yes, these are also identifiable on the lateral projection as well.

Table 5.1
Preferred Appearance by Age of Various Tumors

Age	Benign	Malignant
Infant		Neuroblastoma
3–10	Unicameral bone cyst	Ewing's tumor
	Fibrous cortical defect	
	Localized fibrous dysplasia	
	Benign osteoblastoma	
10–25	Nonossifying fibroma	Osteogenic sarcoma
	Benign chondroblastoma	
	Aneurysmal bone cyst	
20–40	Enchondroma	Reticulum cell sarcoma
	Osteochondroma	Chordoma
	Osteoid osteoma	Fibrosarcoma
	Giant cell tumor	
	Osteoma	
	Chondromyxoid fibroma	
	Hemangioma	
40–70		Chondrosarcoma
		Multiple myeloma
		Metastatic carcinomas

In radiography, the correlation between the clinical, orthopedic, neurological and laboratory findings is paramount in arriving at an appropriate diagnosis. With the possible exception of a blatant fracture, most radiographic indicators are often found in several conditions. This variation of pertinent findings is usually the stumbling block for most students. It causes the greatest degree of confusion and hampers the ability to arrive at a reasonable differential diagnosis.

As one learns to recognize that certain conditions are radiolucent and others are radiopaque and that some present with reactive change and others do not, a certain characteristic form or pattern of presentation occurs for each condition. These patterns of presentation are often quite helpful in the overall recognition of radiographic findings and their subsequent identification.

Additional awareness of these patterns of presentation are enhanced if one is cognizant of the preferred appearance by age, as shown in Table 5.1 above, as well as the preferred characteristics of various bone tumors, as shown in Table 6.1, page 198.

While variations are of course encountered, the information from Tables 5.1 and 6.1 will allow you to form a mental timetable by age of typical presentation and to recognize the frequently encountered characteristics of the various bone tumors. These factors alone will aid you in narrowing down the various options in your differential radiographic diagnosis.

Section 6

Malignant Variations

Case 6.1

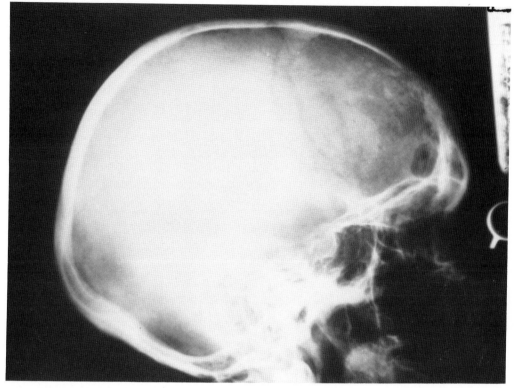

Fig. 6.1A.   Margaret H.

Margaret, a vivacious 68-year-old woman, presented clinically with frequent dull frontal headaches of insidious onset. Examination revealed palpable tenderness with softness over the frontal region of the skull. No neurological deficits were found. Historically, she had had carcinoma of the colon 11 years prior, which had been treated with both surgery and radiation. No recurrence has been reported to date. Laboratory findings included marked elevation of serum alkaline phosphatase with an increase of the A/G ratio and LDH.

A metastatic survey and examination of both the upper and lower gastrointestinal tract were performed, with the only abnormal finding seen in the lateral skull (see Fig. 6.1A).

Is the frontal sinus intact? What is the overall condition of the cortex, skull tables and frontal bone? Is any reactive sclerosis or periosteitis seen?

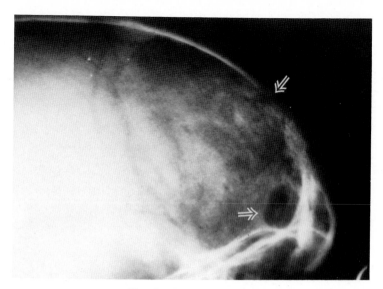

Fig. 6.1*B.*   Margeret H.

The texture of the entire frontal bone is granular in appearance. In your system review, examining the cortex and both outer and inner tables, you find marked loss of continuity (*upper arrow* of Fig. 6.1*B*), indicating bony destruction. No reactive sclerosis or periosteitis is seen, indicating a loss of reparative response. This marked destruction without evidence of repair is characteristic of malignancy. The frontal sinus is intact. The rather large circular area (*lower arrow*) represents loss of substance due to lytic resorption. Other smaller areas of lytic destruction are noted throughout the frontal region.

Metastatic carcinoma from the colon to bone is infrequent but, as in Margaret's case, does occur. As metastatic foci favor the red bone marrow, the most frequent areas of appearance are in the spine, pelvis, ribs, skull, proximal humerus and femur. Metastatic lesions below the elbow and knee are infrequent but do occur, especially with bronchogenic tumors (12).

Case 6.2

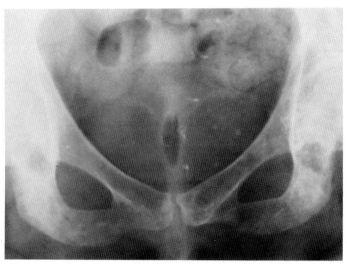

Fig. 6.2A. Nancy L.

Nancy L. is a 40-year-old woman who reports that she has not been feeling well for several months. She "hurts all over." The low back and hips have a constant bony ache. While a 10-pound weight loss has been noticed, she has been dieting and hopes that's the reason. No paresthesias, neuropathy or atrophy has been noted. Bowel and bladder function are normal.

Historically, the patient had had a right radical mastectomy five years prior. Recovery was considered adequate.

After reviewing Fig. 6.2A and other films taken the same day, laboratory tests are ordered. Among these the serum alkaline phosphatase, calcium, and the A/G ratio are abnormal. A moderate leukopenia and hypochromic microcytic anemia are discovered.

Note the architectural structure and texture of the bony matrix. Is there reactive sclerosis or periosteitis? Are there areas of loss of substance, and if so, are these areas well defined with intact margination? How old is the patient?

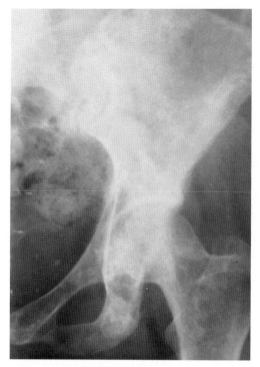

Fig. 6.2*B*.   Nancy L.

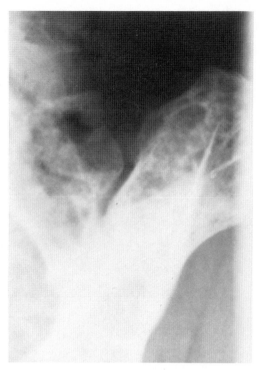

Fig. 6.2*C*.   Nancy L.

Marked loss of substance, disorganized trabecular pattern, the lack of reactive sclerosis or periosteitis, and ill-defined areas of osteolytic destruction are scattered throughout the pubic and ischial rami, as well as the entire right ilium. The oblique view (Fig. 6.2*C*) reveals extensive involvement of the ilium laterally and above the sacroiliac articulation. The cortices are intact but severely thinned. Similar findings have been noted involving the entire pelvis.

The picture of gross *osteolytic metastatic carcinoma from the breast* is derived by history and by labortory and x-ray findings. The most frequent cause of osteolytic metastasis in the child is neuroblastoma;

in an adult male, carcinoma of the lung; and in the adult female, carcinoma of the breast (12).

It is well to remember that pure osteolytic metastasis does not provoke bony proliferation, so a lack of the reparative mechanism is of significance. The process progressively destroys the compacta of bone, thins the cortex and tends towards pathological fracture.

Cartilage is resistant to tumor, thus the intervertebral disc and joint spaces are preserved. This helps differentiate this from an infectious process. The pedicles and body of the vertebrae may be involved. The pedicle involvement helps differentiate from multiple myeloma.

Case 6.3

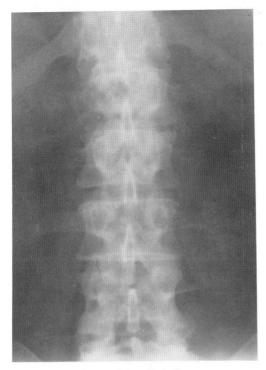

Fig. 6.3A.   Bob O.

Case 6.3 is of an ex-professional football player who had been a patient periodically for years. At 6 foot 4 inches and 265 pounds (he was down from his playing weight), Bob was often asked to do heavy work. He also had occasionally worked as a saloon bouncer.

Usually one or two treatments would suffice to "get his kinks worked out." Bob had reported a "stubborn ache" of his upper lumbar spine for the past two weeks. No other clinical signs were reported. On the day before these films (Fig. 6.3, *A* and *B*) were taken, the dull ache became a sharp, intense pain radiating from the upper lumbar spine around towards the lateral trunk on the left. Moderate muscle splinting was noted. Neurological examination was negative. It was Bob's forty-second birthday.

Within hours after these films were taken, Bob was admitted to the hospital for tests. Mild elevation of serum alkaline phosphatase, LDH and A/G ratio was found. Proteinuria was found, but all kidney function tests were normal.

Two distinct diagnostic possibilities were under consideration based on the films and laboratory tests. The pain became markedly intense over the next 24 hours and permitted surgical entry designed towards nerve decompression. It was of course more exploratory in nature. Once inside, the diagnosis and origin both became evident. Nothing corrective was attempted surgically.

What two probabilities were under consideration based on the above?

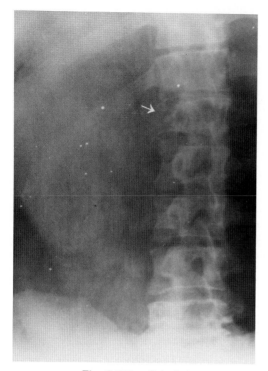

Fig. 6.3B.   Bob O.

Fig. 6.3B, a semioblique lumbar view, was taken immediately after the AP view was seen. Rather marked osteolytic destruction can be seen of the anterolateral section of the L1 vertebral body (see *arrow*). No reactive sclerosis or periosteitis

is present.

The two conditions which were under consideration initially were *metastatic carcinoma* and TB, both of which can cause localized destruction of a vertebral body prior to typical clinical expression.

As mentioned, except for a moderate proteinuria, all kidney function tests were negative. If you will look closely at Fig. 6.3B, you will note an extremely large kidney shadow. This marked enlargement had apparently developed insidiously as an attempt at compensation. At the time Fig. 6.3B was taken, however, function had been totally destroyed, and therefore all measurements and laboratory tests were dealing with the remaining "good" kidney.

Metastatic destruction from the kidney and thyroid, when affecting the peripheral bones, will often present with an expansile, marginated lesion which contains light trabeculation. As the lesion expands, the lesion "blows out" the remaining cortex of bone. This is the so-called "blow out" metastasis. The more central lesion, as in this case, has a much less distinctive appearance than marked osteolytic destruction (12).

Bob refused radiation therapy for the *metastasis from renal carcinoma*, choosing instead to undergo only chemotherapy. After an extremely stormy clinical course, he expired six months later.

Case 6.4

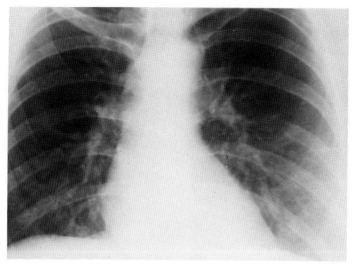

Fig. 6.4A.   Maria T.

Maria is a 46-year-old woman with a history of right mastectomy. This explains the radiolucent lower right lung base (seen in Fig. 6.4A) compared to the left lung base which still has overlying breast tissue.

While the carcinoma had been surgically removed four years prior, Maria has been apprehensive of its return. Over the past two or three months a dull, gnawing pain has been noted at the midthoracic spine, particularly on the left. Last week the pain became sharp, stabbing and constant. She had hoped that she "had a bone out of place." As a slight cough had developed in the last week, the PA chest teleroentgenogram was included in our study. No laboratory work was necessary.

With your careful pattern of review you should be able to identify the lesion. With the history you can put a label on it. Is manipulation indicated?

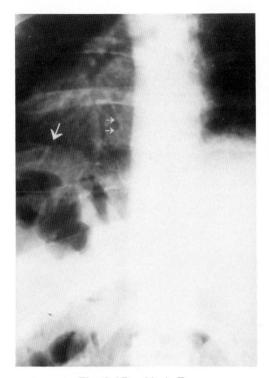
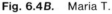

Fig. 6.4*B*. Maria T.

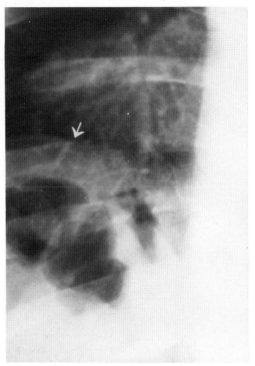

Fig. 6.4*C*. Maria T.

B and *C* of Fig. 6.4 are close-ups of a posterior rib study. At the *large arrow* in both you can identify the blunted end of the remaining seventh posterior rib on the left. The distal portion of the rib is totally destroyed by osteolytic resorption. This represents *osteolytic metastasis from carcinoma of the breast.* No evidence of reactive sclerosis or other reparative mechanisms are seen.

The *small arrows* in Fig. 6.4*B* are directed to the scalloped lateral margin of the sternum—a normal finding—seen also in Fig. 6.4*C*.

The patient was referred for whole-body CT scanning where osteolytic metastasis to the skull was also discovered. Maria expired three months later.

This case is included to exemplify the need for careful, painstaking review of *all* structures on the film. When lesions such as this are not discovered (remember it is just as important when a structure isn't where its supposed to be as when it's an addition to normal), both the patient and the doctor suffer. Manipulation in this instance is definitely contraindicated.

Case 6.5

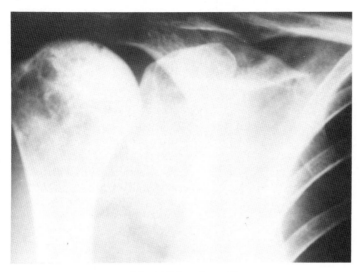

Fig. 6.5A. Anna F.

Anna is a 53-year-old Caucasian woman who presented for examination due to continually worsening bone pain in the left shoulder. Of insidious onset and with intermittent discomfort originally, she thought it would spontaneously abate. It has not. Clinically, the entire humeral head region is tender. Range of motion is guarded but can be performed. An inability to carry, lift or pull with the left shoulder without exacerbation of the pain is reported. Occasional soft-tissue swelling of the shoulder, hand and fingers is noted on the left.

Historically, Anna has had all sorts of problems. Six months ago she underwent radiation therapy for breast carcinoma (on the left). Soon after completion of this she underwent a course of steroid therapy due to a developing arteritis. Her response was considered adequate for both conditions. In case you're wondering, for any JOINT PAIN, Anna always consulted her chiropractor *first*.

The humeral head is of greatest concern. Two simultaneous conditions are present, although it is probable that one precipitated the other—in a roundabout way. This case is semitough, so we'll give a hint. Ever hear of the "snow cap" appearance?

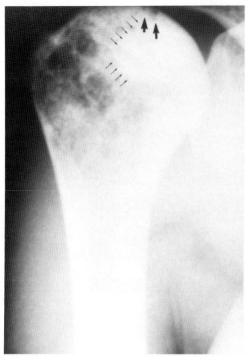

Fig. 6.5B.   Anna F.

The "snow cap" which can be seen in Fig. 6.5, is formed by a dense area of calcification which abuts the joint cortex. It is referred to as an *epiphyseal infarction* and thought by some to be the result of ischemic necrosis (12). Small cortical cystic areas are an early finding, with a thin subcortical band of translucency developing later as the necrosis progresses. Only

the early cystic area can be seen here (see the *arrows* on Fig. 6.5B). As the area loses its blood supply, the bone dies (necrosis) and undergoes softening and fragmentation. In a weight-bearing joint the epiphysis may become deformed. It results from a loss of vascularity from occlusion. While varying etiologies are mentioned, radiation and steroid therapy are both considered likely.

You have undoubtedly noted the multiple areas of loss of substance throughout the greater tubercle and lateral aspect of the head. Thinned cortex is seen, as are disorganization of the matrix and trabecular patterns, and the lack of reparative mechanisms, i.e., reactive sclerosis and periosteitis—a somewhat typical appearance of *osteolytic metastatic carcinoma from the breast.*

In this case the exact etiology of the infarction was never established. It may have been from the radiation or steroid therapy, but it may also have been the result of metastatic invasion. Because the dense sclerotic appearance is generally the result of a reparative response to necrotic bone, we must assume it developed prior to the metastatic bony infiltration.

A note of caution before moving on: The metaphyseal infarctions have a much different appearance, being wedged, serpiginous, clustered, band-like or ring-shaped—definitely unlike the "snow cap" appearance of the epiphyseal lesion.

Case 6.6

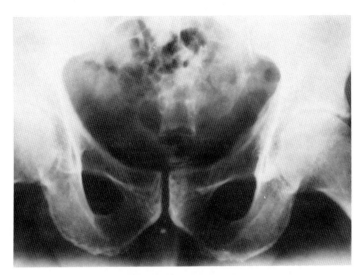

Fig. 6.6A.   Ralph G.

Ralph G. is a 59-year-old man who presented with a dull, bony ache of the low back. He reported that after sitting for prolonged periods he would develop an ache in the groin which seemed to radiate into the low back. No difficulty in urinary function or significant diminution of sexual activity had been noted. Historically, the patient had had prostate surgery eight years prior but was uncertain of the reason. No chemotherapy or radiation treatment followed.

After review of Fig. 6.6A, laboratory tests were done which showed an elevated serum acid phosphatase.

You have probably arrived at a tentative diagnosis already. However, can you identify the radiographic alteration which prompted the laboratory tests?

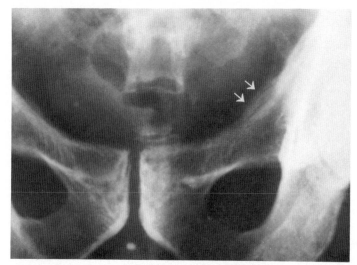

Fib. 6.6*B*.   Ralph G.

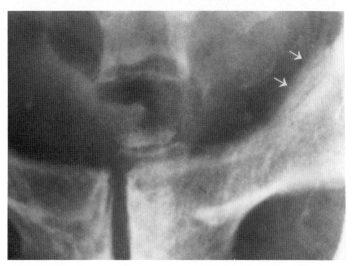

Fig. 6.6*C*.   Ralph G.

You're right again! You noticed the thickened appearance of the pelvic brim on the right. Careful inspection revealed a laminated or "onionskin" appearance of this localized periosteitis (*arrows* in Fig. 6.6, *B* and *C*). Even though you thought Ewing's tumor due to the periosteal appearance, you of course remembered that Ewing's is most often found in patients 15 years of age or under (rarely to age 30). In this patient a metastatic focus was considered. History and clinical findings suggested prostate involvement.

As mentioned, the serum acid phosphatase was elevated, and this localized peri-osteal response was the only bony metastatic focus ever discovered. An unusual and radiographically tough case of *metastatic prostatic carcinoma*.

The unfortunate fact to remember is that in order for the serum acid phosphatase level to be significantly elevated, a breakthrough in the capsule of the prostate must have already occurred. This is often when metastatic spread commences. Newer laboratory techniques are in the development stage which will make possible these determinations of elevation prior to breakthrough of the capsule.

Case 6.7

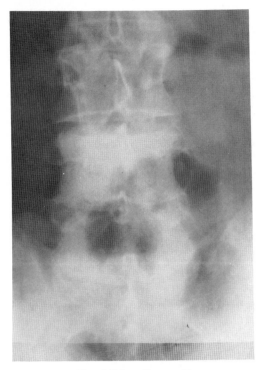

Fig. 6.7A. Barney T.

Barney T. is a 56-year-old Caucasian man who reports progressive increase of bone pain in the lower back.

Orthopedic and neurological testing are essentially unremarkable. No paresthesias or point tenderness is elicited.

Questioning reveals a rapidly declining libido, frequent urination and episodes of incomplete bladder emptying, but no incontinence.

The initial radiograph (Fig. 6.7A) demonstrates a dense sclerotic change with loss of normal architecture involving the L4 vertebral body.

What is the radiolucent shadow covering the inferior portion of the L4 body on the right?

From the history and after review of Fig. 6.7A, a classical pattern of this condition is suspect. Keep in mind that three conditions frequently present with similar radiographic findings. Can you remember all three? What other tests might be required for final determination?

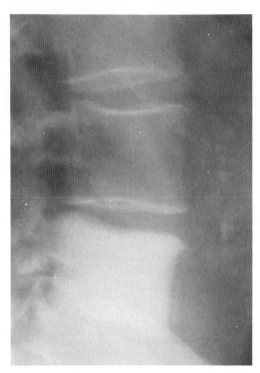

Fig. 6.7B. Barney T.

The three most common conditions which present with dense osteosclerotic change with architectural pattern derangement of the vertebral bodies are osteoblastic metastatic carcinoma of the prostate, Paget's disease and Hodgkin's disease of bone.

The most frequent of these is the *osteoblastic metastasis from the prostate*, as seen in this case (12). It is not unusual to find multiple areas of involvement throughout the lumbar spine and pelvis. In Barney's case, the sole bony lesion is found at L4.

Radiographic differentiation is often difficult but is possible if you recall that in Paget's disease an expansion of bone is noted, giving rise to the "squaring off" of the vertebral margins—the so-called picture frame appearance. The osteosclerosis often has a "softened" appearance and is uniform throughout the affected segments. In Hodgkin's disease, while no pathognomonic radiographic findings are known, the osteosclerotic change is more apt to show spotty areas of osteolytic destruction and will occasionally present with scalloping of the anterior margin of the vertebral body due to pressure erosion by a contiguous lymphadenopathy.

Laboratory differentiation is most useful. Hodgkin's disease will provide various degrees of lymphatic leukemias with associated clinical lymphadenopathy. Paget's disease will record elevated serum alkaline phosphatase, up to ten times normal. In prostatic carcinoma an elevated serum acid phosphatase is found. This recording of elevated acid phosphatase follows breakthrough of the prostate capsule, considered definitive evidence of metastasis.

The radiolucent shadow seen covering the inferior portion of the L4 body on the right in the AP view (Fig. 6.7A) is an overlay of gas. Notice how the shadow extends far beyond the confines of bone.

Case 6.8

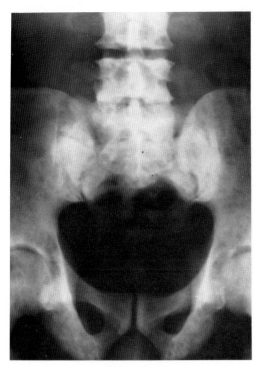

Fig. 6.8*A*.   Frank L.

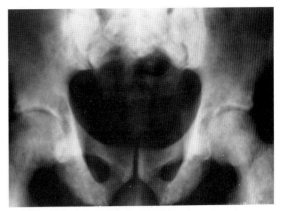

Fig. 6.8*B*.   Frank L.

Frank is a 55-year-old man who reports progressively worsening bone pain of the low back and pelvis. He has lost 20 pounds in the past three months and has the outward appearance of a very cachectic man.

He reports that urinary function is very erratic, and finds incomplete bladder emptying which requires frequent urination. Loss of libido occurred many months ago.

Examination reveals a hard, nodular and enlarged palpable prostate. *A, B* and *C* of Fig. 6.8 confirm your suspicion. There is marked loss of bony detail, multiple small radiolucent lytic lesions scattered throughout, and no evidence of reactive periosteitis or expansion. An overall appearance of increased density of the bony pelvis suggests soft condensation or sclerosis. Indeed, careful review reveals osteolytic destruction surrounded by osteoblastic activity, i.e., a mixed process. The entire pelvis is involved and is also suggested in the lumbar spine. As anticipated, the serum acid phosphatase is markedly elevated—a typical case of *osteoblastic metastasis from prostatic carcinoma.*

Did you also note the neoarthrosis formation on the left, formed by an enlarged transverse process and the sacral ala? This finding of course is architectural and not related to his current problem.

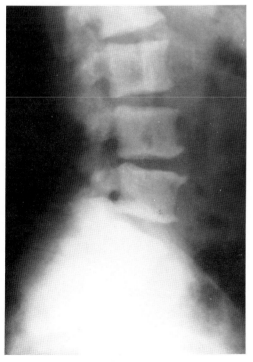

Fig. 6.8*C*.   Frank L.

Case 6.9

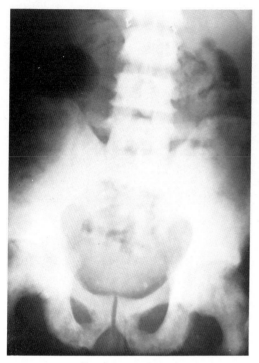

Fig. 6.9A.   Sam J.

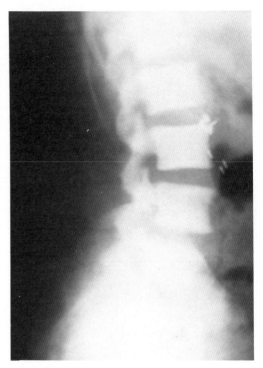

Fig. 6.9B.   Sam J.

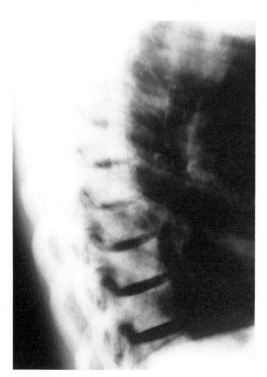

Fig. 6.9C.   Sam J.

A, B, C, D and *E* (Fig. 6.9) are films of Sam taken six months following surgical removal of the prostate. He is currently undergoing chemotherapy and radiation therapy. His prognosis is grave. *A, B, C, D* and *E* are all films of Sam taken the same day. They are included to visually demonstrate the degree of metastasis and the extent of involvement. Gross *osteoblastic activity* is seen in nearly the entire spine. Note the radiographic accentuation of the intervertebral discs in the thoracic spine due to the higher contrast produced by blastic, whitened vertebral bodies. The intervertebral discs have been unaffected, a finding characteristic of metastasis.

The radiopaque metallic densities seen in Fig. 6.9B in the immediate vicinity of the L3 vertebral body are surgical clips and sutures.

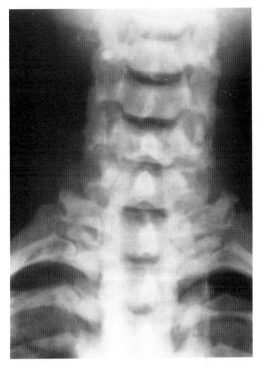

Fig. 6.9D. Sam J.

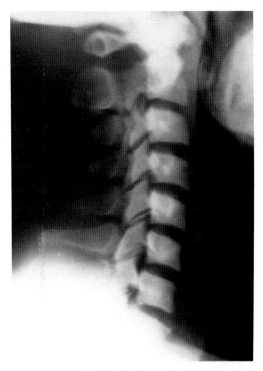

Fig. 6.9E. Sam J.

The cervical films in Sam's case are challenging. The AP view (Fig. 6.9D) reveals a slight mottling of bony texture below C6. Knowing as we do that osteoblastic activity is present in the rest of the spine, it is easy to understand the loss of architectural detail. But what if all we had were these films? Sure makes you want to be certain of good quality films, doesn't it?

The lateral film (Fig. 6.9E) is exciting quality—sharp contrast, great detail—except for one thing. The sharpness is being produced by an overall increase of density within the vertebra. The disc spaces are therefore more accentuated. Notice that the vertebral end plates, which are normally the most radiographically dense part of the bone, are of the same density as the vertebral body. Thus, our supercontrast is being artificially produced by osteoblastic activity within.

Sam's case exemplifies the need for quality films and the painstaking review of all cortical, chondral, periosteal and trabecular patterns when you examine films. It's not just good procedure—it's your professional obligation to the patient.

Table 6.1
Preferred Characteristics of Various Tumors

	Age Group	Sex	Most Frequent Site	Most Frequent Origin	Frequency	Lesion Size
Primary Benign Bone Tumors						
Osteoid osteoma	20–30	Male (2:1)	Femur/tibia		Common	Small
Localized fibrous dysplasia	5–15	Equal	Tibia, skull, pelvis	Metaphysis	Common	Large
Enchondroma	20–50	Equal	Distal metacarpals, proximal phalanges	Metaphysis	Very common	Small
Unicameral bone cyst	3–14	Male (2:1)	Proximal humerus, proximal femur	Metaphysis	Common	Large
Nonossifying fibroma	10–20		Femur/tibia	Metaphysis	Common	Medium
Fibrous cortical defect	4–10	Male	Posterior medial distal femur	Metaphysis	Common	Small
Osteoma	Adult		Frontal/ethmoid sinus, mandible	Intermembranous	Common	Small
Giant cell tumor (quasimalignant)	20–40	Equal	Distal femur, proximal tibia	Metaphysis	Uncommon	Large
Benign chondroblastoma	10–25		Lower femur, upper tibia	Epiphysis	Uncommon	Medium
Aneurysmal bone cyst	10–25		Femur, spine	Metaphysis	Uncommon	Large
Benign osteoblastoma	7–20		Vertebral arch, transverse spinous process, hands, feet	Metaphysis	Rare	Medium
Chondromyxoid fibroma	20–30	Equal	Tibia, femur, pelvis	Metaphysis	Rare	Large
Hemangioma	Adult		Vertebrae, skull		Common	Medium
Osteochondroma (exostosis)	20		Lower femur, upper tibia	Metaphysis	Most common	
Primary Malignant Bone Tumors						
Ewing's tumor	5–30	Equal	Femur, tibia, pelvis	Diaphysis	Common	
Osteogenic sarcoma	10–25	Male (2:1)	Distal femur, proximal tibia	Metaphysis	Common	
Reticulum cell sarcoma	20–40	Male (2:1)	Distal femur, proximal tibia	Diaphysis	Uncommon	
Multiple myeloma	50–70	Male (2:1)	Vertebrae, pelvis, ribs, skull	Diaphysis	Very common	
Chondrosarcoma	40–60	Equal	Femur ends, proximal humerus	Metaphysis	Common	
Fibrosarcoma	25–40	Male (2:1)	Distal femur, proximal tibia	Metaphysis	Rare	
Chordoma	30–70		Sphenoidooccipital sacrococcygeal		Rare	

Most Common Osteolytic Metastases
Child-neuroblastoma
Adult male-carcinoma of lung
Adult female-carcinoma of breast
Most Common Primary Malignant Tumors
1. Multiple myeloma
2. Osteogenic sarcoma
3. Chondrosarcoma

Case 6.10

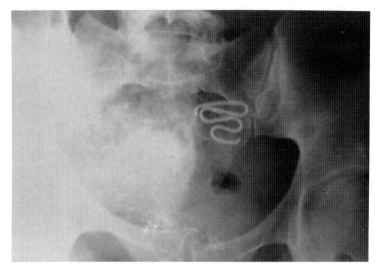

Fig. 6.10A. Susan S.

Susan is a 39-year-old woman who reports low back pain of three months duration with fleeting sciatic irritation on the left. While she denies burning or itching on urination, constipation and painful sexual intercourse have occurred recently. Transient edema of the right ankle and foot is reported.

Examination detects a palpable tender mass within the left intrapelvic region. No abdominal rigidity, localized heat or erythema is detected. Neurologically a loss of pinprick sensation is detected of the L5, S1 and S2 dermatomes. A diminished achilles reflex on the left also is noted.

Laboratory tests reveal an increased serum alkaline phosphatase and calcium levels. All other findings are normal.

Historically, Susan received a "cracked pelvis" following an auto accident many years ago. No recent injuries or illnesses have occurred. The familial history is unrevealing.

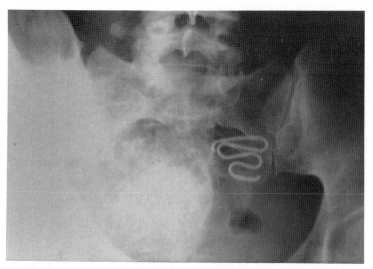

Fig. 6.10B.   Susan S.

Nearly the entire left ilium shows evidence of increased bone density in Fig. 6.10. A dense soft-tissue intrapelvic mass fills the left lower quadrant of the true pelvis. The mass demonstrates with flocculent amorphous and irregular calcification and is, overall, ill-defined. Displacement of neighboring structures is evidenced by right lateral displacement of the intrauterine coil. Destruction of the ilium is not well visualized as yet, but with the degree of sclerotic change it would be probable.

Chondrosarcoma is the third most common primary malignant tumor, following multiple myeloma and osteogenic sarcoma. Two forms are described, the central and the juxtacortical. When originating within the bone it is termed central. When originating outside the confines of the cortex it is considered juxtacortical (12, 23). Susan's case is considered a central form, the most common.

The chondrosarcoma is a malignant tumor of cartilaginous origin. Any bone preformed in cartilage may be involved, but the most frequent sites are the femur and proximal humerus. Characteristically the mass presents with amorphous, punctate, small, flocculent, linear, dense and irregular calcifications. When appearing to radiate from a central point, as in this case, differentiation from an osteogenic sarcoma may be difficult radiographically. While both males and females are about equally affected, chondrosarcoma is usually found in persons over age 40. The osteogenic sarcomas occur most frequently in the early 20s, and multiple myeloma in the late 50s and early 60s. Patient age may be a helpful differential point (see Table 5.1, page 177). Chondrosarcomas are typically slow-growing and metastasize late via the bloodstream (2, 12).

The alteration of the pelvic ring and changes of the pubi seen in Fig. 6.10A are the result of prior trauma and not necessarily related to the chondrosarcoma. On the other hand, a causal relationship between the trauma and malignant degeneration into the chondrosarcoma cannot be ruled out. The neurological variations are due to mass intrusion or pressure deformity.

Case 6.11

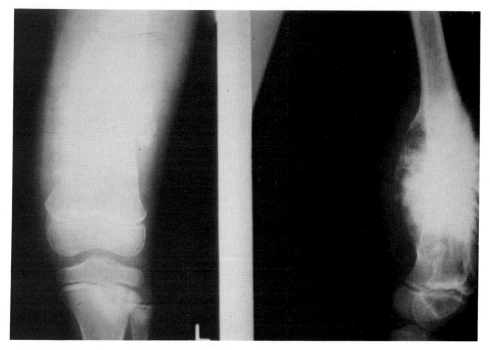

Fig. 6.11. Tabby W.

Tabby is a nine-year-old pixie. About two months ago she complained of pain in her midthigh. Some swelling was noted, but it seemed to dissipate after a few days. Since then, the pain has gradually worsened and the swelling increased.

Examination demonstrates a rather large soft-tissue mass which is tender and nonmovable. No hyperemia is detected, and no effusion of the knee is demonstrated. Tabby reports that she just doesn't feel good. Her mother reports she has had periodic fever over the last few weeks.

Laboratory findings include mild leukocytosis, elevated RBC, sedimentation rate and borderline anemia. The clinical picture simulates acute infectious osteomyelitis, but the time sequence (several months) would indicate another more serious entity.

From Fig. 6.11, the history, and consideration of the clinical presentation and the age of the patient, what do you believe is the most likely diagnosis? Is it benign or malignant?

Case 6.12

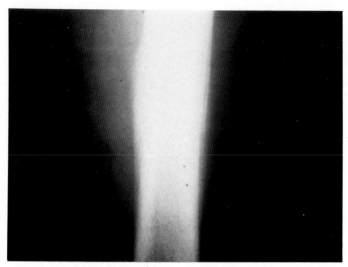

Fig. 6.12. Rick J.

In Fig. 6.12, notice the laminated or "onionskin" appearance of the diaphyseal Ewing's tumor. The soft-tissue swelling is seen surrounding the area. The inner cortex is intact, but the outer margin shows expansion in response to reactive periosteal new bone formation.

Tabby and Rick are both afflicted with *Ewing's tumor.* This primary malignant round cell tumor occurs in persons between 5 and 50 years of age, but it is most frequently seen in children between 10 and 15 years of age. Rick is 14.

The characteristic lesion begins as an area of central destruction within the diaphysis or shaft of the long bones. Due to its origin in bone marrow, younger patients will demonstrate the lesion in the tubular bones, i.e., the femur and tibia, while the favorite site in the older patient (over 20) is the flat bones, i.e., the pelvis. No bone, however, is immune (12).

The lesion presents with an ill-defined area of destruction involving a large central part of the diaphysis. Varying amounts of reactive bone sclerosis are mixed with the osteolysis. After invasion through the cortex, a large fusiform soft-tissue swelling

develops. In an attempt to contain this mass, new periosteal bone formation occurs. With further breakthrough, there is repeated periosteal response. This cyclic destruction-repair mechanism is responsible for the characteristic "onionskin" or laminated periosteal appearance frequently associated with Ewing's tumor. As this laminated appearance occurs in other less malignant lesions, it is not pathognomonic of Ewing's. When seen, however, Ewing's tumor must be ruled out. A soft-tissue mass is invariably present around the lesion. While the laminated or parallel periosteal reaction is typical, slight spiculated response can sometimes be found. There is no "sunburst" from a central point as in osteogenic sarcoma (12, 23).

Typically, Ewing's tumor maintains an intact cortex, albeit expanded, with only segmental destruction. Variable amounts of calcific flecking are seen.

As this is a tumor of bone marrow, metastasis via direct extension or hematogenous spread is rapid. The prognosis is poor. (Both Tabby and Rick expired within one year of discovery of the lesion).

Case 6.13

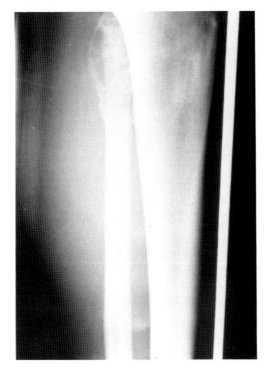

Fig. 6.13A. Randy S.

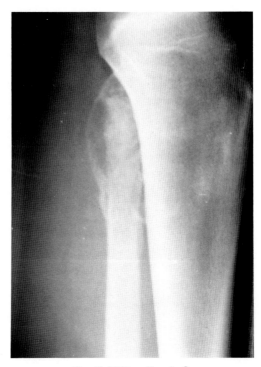

Fig. 6.13B. Randy S.

Randy is a 20-year-old man who developed painful swelling just below his right knee. He reports that when it first began about eight weeks ago, he thought he had bruised it. Slight swelling appeared and has progressively worsened. The patient is afebrile, although the swollen area demonstrates with mild hyperemia. The knee is capable of full range of motion in the non-weight-bearing state. With weight bearing, moderate pain is noted over the palpable mass located at the end of the proximal fibula.

Laboratory results indicate mild elevation of the serum alkaline phosphatase. The WBC count and the sedimentation rate are normal.

A and *B* of Fig. 6.13 indicate an expanding metaphyseal lesion of the proximal fibula, immediately below the fused epiphyseal plate. Reactive periosteitis is noted with a moderate-sized soft-tissue mass surrounding the lesion. Amorphous calcific streaking also is noted, extending laterally from the medial margin of the lesion, overlying the proximal tibia. A dense sclerotic thickening of the proximal fibular shaft obscures the medullary cavity.

With the rather prolonged lead time, lack of systemic fever and normal WBC count, osteomyelitis can be ruled out. Remembering the age of the patient, do you have a suggested diagnosis for this expanding, destructive lesion?

Case 6.13 *continued*   # Case 6.14

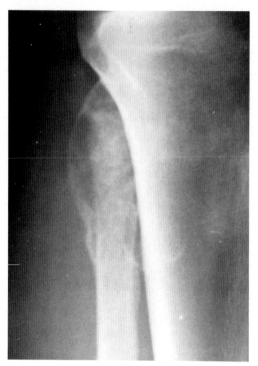

Fig. 6.13C.   Randy S.

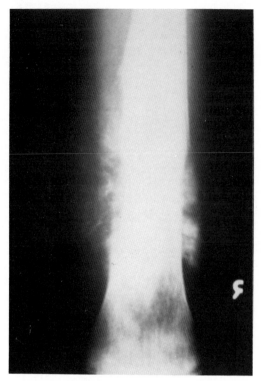

Fig. 6.14.   Tina B.

Osteogenic sarcoma is the second most common primary malignant tumor of bone. Multiple myeloma is the most common. The majority of osteogenic sarcomas occur in males (2:1) in the 10- to 25-year age bracket. Generally, in the younger patient the tubular bones are involved, whereas in the older patient, the flat bones are the favored sites. The most frequent sites of the central osteosarcoma are the distal femur and proximal tibia (12). (Other types, which will not be dealt with here, are the parosteal, multiple sarcomatosis and the soft-tissue sarcoma. Each has differing clinical findings and prognosis.)

The tumor is fast-growing with an early incidence of pulmonary metastasis via the bloodstream. The prognosis is poor. Usually in the tubular bones the lesion begins in the metaphysis. If occurring after epiphyseal closure, the epiphysis is commonly involved.

Radiographically the lesion may appear as a dense sclerosis, as an admixture of ossifying and lytic destruction or, less frequently, as purely osteolytic. The predominant feature is the reactive periosteal response. While a laminated appearance is frequent, as in Randy's case, the "sunburst" pattern resulting from radiating spiculation from a central point is better known (see Fig. 6.14). With expansion of the lesion and the attempt at repair by the periosteum, an elevation or triangle known as Codman's triangle may develop. As the lesion breaks through the cortex, invasion into soft tissue occurs. Amorphous calcification surrounds the sarcomatous spicules into the tumor and appears to be extending from the centrum of the lesion, i.e., "sunburst."

(In Randy's case, amputation was done above the knee, and eight years later he's doing fine—a somewhat rare happening. Tina was 17 years old when the lesion shown in Fig. 6.14 was discovered in a more typical location, i.e., the distal femur. Metastasis to the lung had already occurred, and she expired eight months later.)

Case 6.15

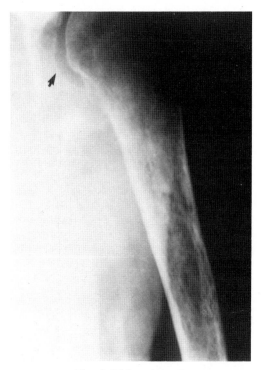

Fig. 6.15A.   John B.

Mr. B. is a 78-year-old gentleman. A retired naval officer, his appearance and demeanor belie his age.

He reports that for the past two months it has become nearly impossible for him to abduct his left arm without pain into the shoulder. He notices some extension of "muscle ache" extending down the outside of the upper arm into the lateral elbow. No significant history of accident or illness is discovered, although he reports that he did notice periodic ache of the shoulder-arm following a week of golf tournaments a few months prior. Orthopedic examination demonstrates marked limitation of shoulder excursion (the arc of painful movement limiting abduction to 50° to 55°), moderate loss of pinwheel sensation over both radial and ulnar distribution peripherally, and loss of grip strength and tactile sensation on the left. At the time films were taken, laboratory tests were ordered.

Mr. B. was very upset with us when we failed to institute immediate treatment for his "bursitis."

Before turning the page, notice the marked derangement of the glenoid fossa in Fig. 6.15A. Bony destruction is evident with a lack of reactive sclerosis or periosteitis. No subchondral cyst-like areas of degenerative joint disease are seen, and the remaining articular joint space appears widened by the destruction.

Results from which particular laboratory test would you be most anxious to see?

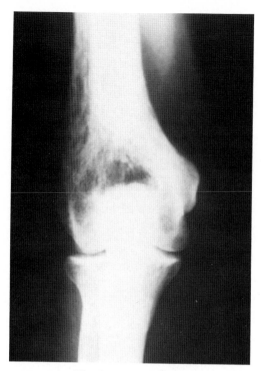

Fig. 6.15B. John B.

We were extremely anxious to have the results of the serum alkaline phosphatase, acid phosphatase, calcium, A/G ratio and protein electrophoresis. For old times sake we also ordered a Bence-Jones (B-J) protein urine determination.

The results of our tests indicated an elevated calcium level and reversed A/G ratio, and the electrophoretic study indi-cated a hyperglobulinemia. The Bence-Jones was negative (not surprising in that only about 40% of tests show detectable B-J proteinuria by the heating method (12)).

Notice the rather diffuse loss of bone density throughout the humerus in Fig. 6.15, *A* and *B*. Disorganization and altera-tion of bone texture are seen. Multiple, small *punched-out* areas of osteolytic de-struction permeate the midshaft and tend to coalesce into larger areas of loss of substance. Trabecular patterns are lacking, and marked thinning of the cortex is pres-ent. When these observations were cou-pled with the laboratory findings, a diag-nosis of *multiple myeloma* was made.

The hallmark radiographic findings in multiple myeloma are the multiple, sharply circumscribed, punched-out le-sions. Without this permeative pattern, the osteolytic destruction is very much like that of osteolytic metastases.

Because the loss of bone density results from a diffuse marrow involvement with myeloma tissue, the inner margin of the cortex is frequently involved, producing scalloping of the endosteum (see Fig. 6.15*A*).

Multiple myeloma is a primary malig-nant tumor of bone marrow. It is the most common primary malignant neoplasm in-volving bone. It is rare under the age of 30 years, with the vast majority of patients being between 50 and 70 years of age. Males are affected twice as often as fe-males.

Case 6.16

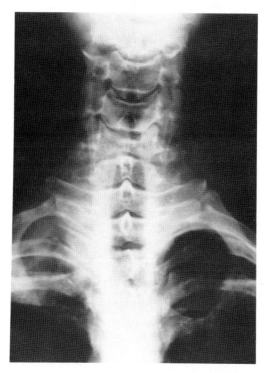

Fig. 6.16A. Jack B.

Jack is a 44-year-old man who was persuaded by his wife to come in after the pain and weakness in his left arm became so bad that he cancelled two golf dates in one week (now that's bad!).

Jack relates that for the past eight to ten weeks he has had progressive weakness and pain in his left shoulder, arm and hand. Two weeks ago he noticed his watch band becoming loose and wondered if he was losing weight. Soon after, the upper eyelid of his left eye began to sag and was commented on by other people. Early this week he noticed pain and ache at the base of his neck, extending into the shoulder and anterior chest.

Neurological examination reveals diminished deep tendon reflex of the left upper extremity, loss of tactile, tensile and grip of the left hand, contraction of the left pupil and loss of ciliospinal reflex.

At that time, radiography was done, and on the basis of clinical and x-ray findings a diagnosis was made. No laboratory tests were ordered.

From the above description and Fig. 6.16A, can you provide a working diagnosis? Let me give you a hint—it's a classic textbook case with no tricks, and it all fits. How will you treat this patient?

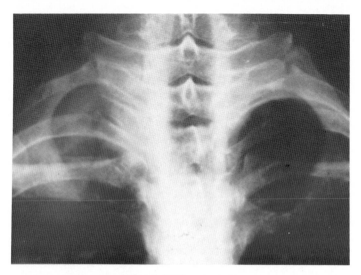

Fig. 6.16B.   Jack B.

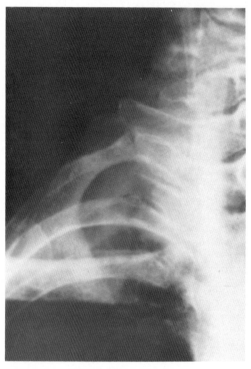

Fig. 6.16C.   Jack B.

In your review of *all* the structures on the film, Fig. 6.16*A*, you undoubtedly noticed the marked variation in density of the lung apices. The left apex contains a definite mass. Close observation will also reveal osteolytic resorption of part of the second posterior rib on the left (Fig. 6.16, *B* and *C*).

The four cardinal parts of the Pancoast syndrome are a mass in the pulmonary apex, destruction of adjacent rib or vertebra, Horner's syndrome and pain down the arm (23). In Jack's case all criteria are met, and this is indeed a *Pancoast tumor.*

The Pancoast tumor is a superior pulmonary sulcus tumor usually caused by a squamous cell type of bronchogenic tumor. When the mass interferes with the sympathetic fibers of the first thoracic ganglion, it affects the entire one half of the face, producing Horner's syndrome of enophthalmos, drooping of the upper eyelid, contraction of the pupil and absence of sweating in the entire upper extremity, all unilaterally (20).

Radiation therapy in Jack's case was successful in shrinking the tumor. Some slow reversal of other symptoms has occurred and is continuing.

Case 6.17

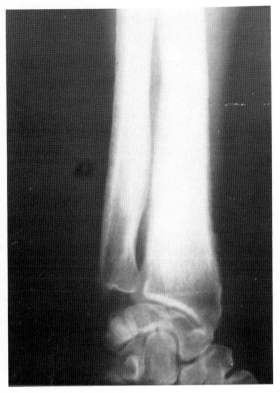

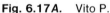

Fig. 6.17A.   Vito P.

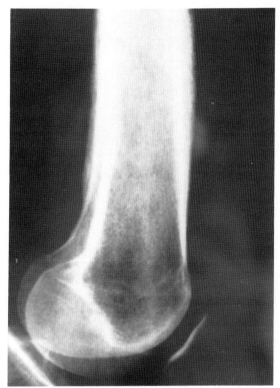

Fig. 6.17B.   Vito P.

Vito P. is a 38-year-old man who presented with multiple joint pains of long standing. He reported generalized weakness, easy fatigability and frequent dyspnea. Symptoms had come on gradually. When he noticed that the discomfort in his knees and elbows had not eased with rest, he became concerned. Also, he reported a curious change in the size and shape of the ends of his fingers. His fingernails seemed to be growing down over the ends of the fingertips. A bluish discoloration of the nail beds would occasionally appear.

Vito indicated that he had had transient soft-tissue swelling of the elbows, knees and ankles. It had usually gone away spontaneously, and although the joint pain con-

tinued, he was not compelled to seek help. He also indicated that his smoker's cough has worsened lately, but he thought it was the result of having a cold or sinus drainage.

Examination revealed palpable tenderness over the entire femur, knee, forearm and wrist. Slight tissue edema was suspect. Neurological and orthopedic testing were inconclusive. Auscultory examination indicated slight wheezing sounds of the right upper lung field. The apices were bilaterally clear. Running in place caused dyspnea. Blood pressure was 136/80; pulse rate, 74. Carotid bruits were not demonstrated. The x-rays, of which *A* and *B* appear above, were near definitive—any ideas?

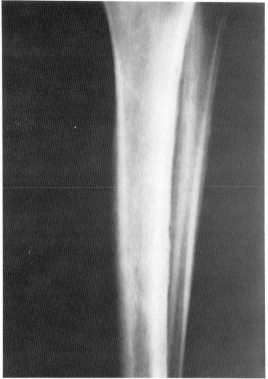

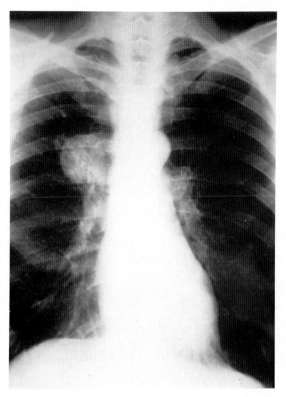

Fig. 6.17C.   Vito P.

Fig. 6.17D.   Vito P.

The triad of clubbing of the fingers, periosteal new bone formation of the shafts of the cylindrical bones of the extremities, and a type of joint arthropathy is referred to as the syndrome of *pulmonary hypertrophic osteoarthropathy.* As experience has shown that the condition can also occur in conditions other than those associated with the thorax, the term pulmonary is now dropped by some authors (2). Little doubt remains that the condition is most often associated with pulmonary neoplasm, chronic tuberculosis, empyema, bronchiectasis and abscess.

Radiographically, periosteal new bone can be seen formed along the outer surface of the diaphysis of tubular bones. It may blend with the cortex, causing a thickening of same. Occasionally a thin radiolucent line (Fig. 6.17C) may be seen separating the periosteum from the cortex. This line represents the fibrous matrix where the new bone is first formed. Periosteal response typically has a shaggy or roughened appearance. The ends of bone are not involved.

In Vito's case the chest teleroentgenogram clearly defined a bronchogenic neoplasm in the right lung (Fig. 6.17D). Complete disappearance of the osteoarthropic signs and symtoms has occurred following total ablation of the pulmonary lesion (18).

References

1. Aegerter, E., and Kirkpatrick, Jr., J.A.: Arthritis. In *Orthopedic Diseases*, ed. 4. W.B. Saunders Company, Philadelphia, 1975.
2. Aegerter, E., and Kirkpatrick, Jr., J.A.: Circulatory Disturbances. In *Orthopedic Diseases*, ed. 4. W.B. Saunders Company, Philadelphia, 1975.
3. Copeland, M.M., and Geschickter, C.F.: Cartilaginous tumors of bone. In *M.D. Anderson Hospital and Tumor Institute: Tumors of Bone and Soft Tissue*, pp. 279–298. Year Book Medical Publishers, Chicago, 1965.
4. Dolan, K.D.: Expanding lesions of the cervical spine canal. *Radiol. Clin. North Am.*, 15(2): 203–214, 1977.
5. Epstein, B., Epstein, J., and Jones, M.D.: Cervical spinal stenosis. *Radiol. Clin. North Am.*, 15(2): 215–225, 1977.
6. Epstein, B., Epstein, J., and Jones, M.D.: Lumbar spinal stenosis. *Radiol. Clin. North Am.*, 15(2): 227–239, 1977.
7. Fardon, D.F.: Odontoid fracture complicating ankylosing hyperostosis of the spine. *Spine*, 3(2): 108–112, 1978.
8. Fenlin, J.M.: Pathology of degenerative disease of the cervical spine. *Orthop. Clin. North Am.*, 2(2): 371–387, 1971.
9. Finneson, B.E.: Lumbar disc disease. In *Low Back Pain*, ed. 2. J.B. Lippincott Company, Philadelphia, 1980.
10. Forestier, J., and Lagier, R.: Ankylosing hyperostosis of the spine. *Clin. Orthop.*, 74: 65–83, 1971.
11. Forrester, D.M., and Nesson, J.W.: Arthritis from head to foot. In *The Radiology of Joint Disease*. W.B. Saunders Company, Philadelphia, 1973.
12. Greenfield, G.B.: The cardinal roentgen features. In *Radiology of Bone Diseases*. J.B. Lippincott Company, Philadelphia, 1969.
13. Greenfield, G.B.: The solitary lesion. In *Radiology of Bone Diseases*. J.B. Lippincott Company, Philadelphia, 1969.
14. Grobler, L.J., Simmons, E.H., and Varrington, T.W.: International disc herniation in the adolescent. *Spine*, 4(3): 267–278, 1979.
15. Hildebrandt, R.W.: Pelvic and spinal biomechanics. In *Chiropractic Spinography*. Hilmark Publications, Des Plaines, Ill., 1977.
16. Hutton, W.C., Scott, J.R.R., and Cyron, B.M.: Is spondylolysis a fatigue fracture? *Spine*, 2(3): 202–209, 1977.
17. McAlister, W.H., and Shackelford, G.D.: Measurement of spinal curvatures. *Radiol. Clin. North Am.*,13(1): 113–121, 1975.
18. Martel, W.: Radiology of the rheumatic diseases. *JAMA*, 224(5): 69: 129–136, 1973.
19. Meschan, I.: Radiology of joints. In *Analysis of Roentgen Signs in General Radiology*, vol. 1. W.B. Saunders Company, Philadelphia, 1973.
20. Meschan, I.: Radiology of the vertebral column. In *Roentgen Signs in Clinical Practice*, vol. 1. W.B. Saunders Company, Philadelphia, 1966.
21. Moe, J.H., Winter, R.B., Bradford, D.S., and Longstein, J.E.: Radiographic evaluation. In *Scoliosis and Other Spinal Deformities*, pp. 31–40. W.B. Saunders Company, Philadelphia, 1978.
22. Paul, L.W., and Juhl, J.H.: Diseases of the joints. In *The Essentials of Roentgen Interpretation*, ed. 3. Harper & Row, Hagerstown, Md., 1972.
23. Paul, L.W., and Juhl, J.H.: Miscellaneous conditions. In *The Essentials of Roentgen Interpretation*, ed. 3. Harper & Row, Hagerstown, Md., 1972.
24. Wiltse, L.L.: The effect of the common anomalies of the lumbar spine upon disc degeneration and low back pain. *Orthop. Clin. North Am.*, 2(2): 569–582, 1971.
25. White III, A.A., and Panjabi, M.M.: The clinical biomechanics of spine pain. In *Clinical Biomechanics of the Spine*. J.B. Lippincott Company, Philadelphia, 1978.
26. White III, A. A., and Panjabi, M. M.: Physical properties and functional biomechanics of the spine. In *Clinical Biomechanics of the Spine*. J. B. Lippincott Company, Philadelphia, 1978.
27. LaRocca, H.: New horizons in research on disc disease. *Orthop. Clin. North Am.*, 2(2): 521–531, 1971.
28. Rothman, R.H.: The clinical syndrome of lumbar disc disease. *Orthop. Clin. North Am.*, 2(2): 463–476, 1971.
29. Maurer, E.L.: The thoraco-costal facet syndrome with introduction of the marginal line and the rib sign. *ACA J. Chiropractic*, 13(12): vol. X, 5–151–164, 1976.
30. Zohn, D.A., and Mennell, J.M.: Crossmatching clinical diagnosis with treatment principles. In *Musculoskeletal Pain: Diagnosis and Physical Treatment*, Little, Brown & Company, Boston, 1976.
31. Gehweiler, Jr., J.A., Osborne, Jr., R.L., and Becker, R.F.: Spondylolisthesis without spondylolysis. In *The Radiology of Vertebral Trauma*. W.B. Saunders Company, Philadelphia, 1980.
32. Cyron, B.M., and Hutton, W.C.: Articular tropism and stability of the lumbar spine. *Spine*, 5(2): 168–172, 1980.

Supplemental Reading

Cyriax, J.: *Textbook of Orthopaedic Medicine*, vol. 1., ed. 6. Bailliére Tindall, London, 1975.

Farfan, H.F., and Sullivan, J.D.: The relation of facet orientation to intervertebral disc failure. *Can. J. Surg.*, 10: 179, 1967.

Hadley, L.A.: *Anatomic Roentgenographic Studies of the Spine*, ed. 2. Charles C Thomas Company, Springfield, Ill., 1973.

MacGibbon, B., and Farfan, H.F.: A radiologic survey of various configurations of the lumbar spine. *Spine*, 4(3): 258–266, 1979.

Madewell, J., Ragsdale, B.D., and Sweet, D.E.: Radiologic and pathologic analysis of solitary bone lesions, Part I: Internal margins. *Radiol. Clin. North. Am.*, 19(4): 715–748, 1981.

Malcolm, B.W.: Spinal deformity secondary to spinal injury. *Orthop. Clin. North Am.*, 10(4): 943–952, 1979.

Marvel, Jr., J.P.: The clinical syndrome of cervical disc disease. *Orthop. Clin. North Am.*, 2(2): 419–433, 1971.

Maurer, E.L.: Arthrosis—what's in a name? *Success Express*, 4: 4, 1981.

Maurer, E.L.: The periosteum. *Success Express*, 5(1): 27–32, 1982.

Ragsdale, B.D., Madewell, J.E., and Sweet, D.E.: Radiologic and pathologic analysis of solitary bone lesions, Part II: Periosteal reactions. *Radiol. Clin. North Am.*, 19(4): 749–783, 1981.

Rosse, C., and Clawson, D.K.: *The Musculoskeletal System in Health and Disease.* Harper & Row, Hagerstown, Md., 1980.

Rothman, R.H., and Simeone, F.A.: *The Spine*, vols. I and II. W.B. Saunders Company, Philadelphia, 1975.

Sweet, D.B., Madewell, J.E., and Ragsdale, B.D.: Radiologic and pathologic analysis of solitary bone lesions, Part III: Matrix patterns. *Radiol. Clin. North Am.*, 19(4): 785–814, 1981.

Schutta, H.S., and Elliott, F.A.: The differential diagnosis of sciatica. *Orthop. Clin. North Am.*, 2(2): 477–484, 1971.

Index